100 Questions & Answers About Lung Cancer

Second Edition

Joan H. Schiller, MD

Professor and Chief, Division of Hematology and Oncology
Deputy Director of Simmons Comprehensive Cancer Center
Andrea L. Simmons Distinguished Chair in Cancer Research
University of Texas Southwestern Medical Center
President, National Lung Cancer Partnership
Dallas, Texas

Karen Parles, MLS

Editor, LungCancerOnline

Amy Cipau, MBA

President, Board Member
North Carolina Lung Cancer Partnership
Raleigh, North Carolina

JONES AND BARTLETT PUBLISHERS
Sudbury, Massachusetts
BOSTON   TORONTO   LONDON   SINGAPORE

616.994
SCH

World Headquarters

Jones and Bartlett Publishers
40 Tall Pine Drive
Sudbury, MA 01776
978-443-5000
info@jbpub.com
www.jbpub.com

Jones and Bartlett Publishers
Canada
6339 Ormindale Way
Mississauga, Ontario L5V 1J2
Canada

Jones and Bartlett Publishers
International
Barb House, Barb Mews
London W6 7PA
United Kingdom

Jones and Bartlett's books and products are available through most bookstores and online booksellers. To contact Jones and Bartlett Publishers directly, call 800-832-0034, fax 978-443-8000, or visit our website www.jbpub.com.

Substantial discounts on bulk quantities of Jones and Bartlett's publications are available to corporations, professional associations, and other qualified organizations. For details and specific discount information, contact the special sales department at Jones and Bartlett via the above contact information or send an email to specialsales@jbpub.com.

The authors, editor, and publisher have made every effort to provide accurate information. However, they are not responsible for errors, omissions, or for any outcomes related to the use of the contents of this book and take no responsibility for the use of the products and procedures described. Treatments and side effects described in this book may not be applicable to all people; likewise, some people may require a dose or experience a side effect that is not described herein. Drugs and medical devices are discussed that may have limited availability controlled by the Food and Drug Administration (FDA) for use only in a research study or clinical trial. Research, clinical practice, and government regulations often change the accepted standard in this field. When consideration is being given to use of any drug in the clinical setting, the healthcare provider or reader is responsible for determining FDA status of the drug, reading the package insert, and reviewing prescribing information for the most up-to-date recommendations on dose, precautions, and contraindications, and determining the appropriate usage for the product. This is especially important in the case of drugs that are new or seldom used.

Production Credits

Executive Publisher: Christopher Davis
Custom Projects Editor: Kathy Richardson
Senior Editorial Assistant: Jessica Acox
Production Director: Amy Rose
Production Editor: Daniel Stone

Marketing Manager: Ilana Goddess
V.P. of Manufacturing and Inventory Control:
   Therese Connell
Composition: Spoke & Wheel/Jason Miranda
Printing and Binding: Malloy, Inc.

Cover Credits

Cover Design: Carolyn Downer
Cover Image: Top left photo: © absolut/ShutterStock, Inc., Top right photo: © Melissa Brandes/ShutterStock, Inc.,
   Bottom Photo: © Rob Marmion/ShutterStock, Inc.
Cover Printing: Malloy, Inc.

Library of Congress Cataloging-in-Publication Data

Schiller, J. H. (Joan H.), 1954-
   100 questions & answers about lung cancer / Joan Schiller, Karen Parles, Amy Cipau. — 2e.
      p. cm.
   Parles' name appears first on the earlier edition.
   Includes bibliographical references and index.
   ISBN-13: 978-0-7637-6053-3
   ISBN-10: 0-7637-6053-6
   1. Lungs—Cancer—Popular works. I. Parles, Karen. II. Cipau, Amy. III. Title. IV. Title: 100 questions and answers about lung cancer. V. Title: One hundred questions and answers about lung cancer.
   RC280.L8P365 2009
   616.99'424—dc22

                              2009007079
6048

Printed in the United States of America
13 12 11 10 09   10 9 8 7 6 5 4 3 2 1

Dedicated to Karen Parles.

After an eleven-year struggle with non-small cell lung cancer, Karen passed away on February 16, 2009. She dedicated her life and her energies to the well-being of her family and friends, and to improving the quality of care and information provided to people living with lung cancer. Thanks, in part, to Karen, lung cancer patients now receive greater respect as well as better information about their illness, and lung cancer research is more appropriately funded.

Her strength and courage have inspired thousands.

CONTENTS

Part 10: If Treatment Fails   **175**

Part 11: Prevention, Screening, and Advocacy   **185**

When I was asked by Karen Parles, Amy Cipau, and Joan Schiller to write the Foreword to the first edition of *100 Questions & Answers About Lung Cancer*, I was honored to say yes, and now I am pleased to have that opportunity again with the second edition of this valuable book.

Lung cancer, the most common cause of cancer death in the United States, killing more people every year than breast, colon, and prostate cancers combined, is a neglected and under-reported disease. A media survey commissioned by Cancer*Care* in 2005, reviewing 600 news stories about cancer, confirmed some progress in attention to lung cancer over our 2000 analysis. However, there were still fewer broadcast, print, and online stories than the three other major cancers. There continue to be few celebrities, few events, few first-person stories, and little attention to progress in detection or treatment of lung cancer. Much coverage of lung cancer is still directed at tobacco being its primary cause.

I have spent my professional life of more than 30 years working in the field of cancer, and I am well aware that "competition" among diseases is not productive for patients, clinicians, or researchers. However, it's clearly time to intensify our focus on lung cancer and provide education, support, and increased research funding to this disease. Lung cancer remains the cancer that is stigmatized, with a "blame the victim" attitude. This perception, often held by the lay public and many professionals, can lead to isolation for people coping with this illness and frequently prevents them from understanding treatment options. It is crucial that people diagnosed with lung cancer know that they have the right to seek information, ask questions, and have a clear understanding of the choices available. A book such as this one gives the patient and family crucial information and support that they need to cope at a time of anxiety and confusion. Karen, Amy, and Joan are leaders in their respective fields, and the experience and knowledge that they bring provides an outstanding resource for anyone concerned about lung cancer. They represent just what we need to help those with lung cancer: experienced, knowledgeable individuals who are ready to speak out about this disease.

As Executive Director of Cancer*Care*, I have had the opportunity to develop support and education services for people with lung cancer. Cancer*Care* offers professional counseling, telephone and online support groups for patients and caregivers, telephone education workshops, publications, financial assistance, and practical help completely free of charge to people with lung cancer and their loved ones. Karen Parles, Amy Cipau, and Joan Schiller are committed advocates and professionals who want to seize this moment and add their articulate voices to the knowledge of lung cancer. *100 Questions & Answers About Lung Cancer, Second Edition,* is a cornerstone of our efforts to have an impact on this difficult disease; it enables patients and families to seek out the best treatment with the goal of the best possible outcome. Progress is being made in detection and treatment of lung cancer. We need to get that word out, and Karen, Amy, and Joan are experts who are using their extensive experience to provide accurate information, support, and, importantly, hope to the tens of thousands of people coping with lung cancer.

Armed with this book, no one with lung cancer needs be alone in the fight against the disease. Use it as an information source, seek support, ask questions; you have a wonderful resource available to you right here.

Diane Blum, MSW
Executive Director of Cancer*Care*
New York, NY

Lung cancer today is not the same disease it was 20 years ago, or even (six) years ago, when this book was first published. Over the last several years, new treatments for lung cancer have been developed and tested. New surgical techniques that cause less pain and shorter recoveries have become more widely available. New radiation-focusing devices ensure that only the tumor, and not the healthy tissue surrounding it, gets treated. Additional chemotherapy agents and targeted therapies—medicines designed to specifically attack cancer cells—have brought new hope to the people diagnosed with this disease and their families.

This book provides an overview of lung cancer for the person looking for a deeper understanding of what it is, and how to cope with the diagnosis, as well as side effects of treatment. Receiving a lung cancer diagnosis can be scary and life-changing, but a key part of living with lung cancer is to learn the facts, and stay positive and hopeful. This book is designed to answer some of the most common questions patients and their loved ones may have, while also providing sources for additional information.

The information in this book will also help you understand how important it is to take an active role in making treatment-related decisions. A very significant decision for anyone entering lung cancer treatment is to consider whether participating in a clinical trial is right for them. Those who participated in clinical trials in the past have made possible the treatment advances of today. Further advances, and someday cures, cannot happen unless patients get involved in clinical research. If you are interested in taking part in a clinical trial and your doctor does not discuss this option with you, ask whether there may be an opportunity for you to participate.

Most importantly, perhaps, this book lets you know that you are not alone. There are over 200,000 Americans diagnosed with lung cancer each year, so there are peers for you to speak with and support groups to lean on. Talk to your doctor, nurse or social worker, and call Cancer*Care* (1-800-813-HOPE) to find out about support networks available to you.

The progress that has been made in understanding the disease has been immense, but there is still a tremendous amount we do not know about lung cancer. Dr. Schiller and her colleagues founded the National Lung Cancer Partnership (*www.NationalLungCancerPartnership.org*) to increase the amount of funding available for lung cancer research, and to raise awareness that lung cancer can happen to anyone: young or old, male or female, smoker, former smoker, or never smoker. We are working to empower patients so they can make the best possible treatment choices, educate doctors to increase their ability to diagnose the disease earlier and provide the best available treatments, and raise awareness among the public to dispel the notion that this disease is "self-inflicted" and therefore unworthy of support. We also directly fund lung cancer research, and train advocates to raise the profile of lung cancer in their communities, in an effort to increase the level of funding for this disease.

Other cancers have seen great strides in awareness, and consequently research funding. For example, successes in breast cancer screening, treatment and care came about because devoted, caring people joined together to raise awareness of the disease and funds for research. We need the same for lung cancer. We need people who have been affected by lung cancer to tell their stories, write to their congressional representatives, and work to raise awareness of and research funding for lung cancer. National Lung Cancer Partnership's *Free to Breathe*™ lung cancer awareness event series (*www.FreetoBreathe.org*) is designed around this need; the numbers of events and participants are growing each year, bringing greater attention to this challenging disease in local communities.

By reading this book, you'll have taken the first step toward understanding this disease. When you arm yourself with knowledge about lung cancer, you enable yourself to take charge of your care and your life.

Regina Vidaver, PhD
Executive Director
National Lung Cancer Partnership

PART ONE

The Basics

What is cancer?

What should I know about cancer cells?

How do normal lungs function?

More . . .

Cells

Microscopic units that make up the organs of the body.

Cancer cells differ from normal cells in a number of important ways. First, they are often unable to stop growing and dividing ("unregulated growth"). Second, cancer cells often stop "doing their thing." In fact, they often stop doing anything useful at all.

White blood cells

A type of blood cell which fights infection.

Apoptosis

Process by which normal cells die when they are injured; often referred to as "programmed cell death."

Metastasis

The spread of cancer from the initial cancer site to other parts of the body.

1. What is cancer?

Cancer is uncontrolled growth of **cells**—the billions upon billions upon billions of microscopic units that make up all the organs of our body. Cells are easily distinguished from each other: lung cells are very different in appearance from colon cells, and do very different things. They are very different from blood cells, which are very different from muscle cells, and so forth. To understand what cancer is, you must first understand what makes a normal cell "normal."

Normal cells "do their own thing." For example, red blood cells carry oxygen throughout the body, stomach cells absorb nutrients, and **white blood cells** fight infections. Normal cells also stop growing and dividing when they get too old. In addition, normal cells often "self destruct" (undergo **apoptosis**) and die if they are injured.

Cancer cells differ from normal cells in a number of important ways. First, they are often unable to stop growing and dividing ("unregulated growth"). Second, cancer cells often stop "doing their thing." In fact, they often stop doing anything useful at all. For example, cancerous white blood cells often stop fighting infection, stomach cancer cells stop absorbing nutrients, and lung cancer cells are unable to absorb oxygen. Another property of cancer cells is that they do not die like normal cells do when they grow old; they are literally immortal. In addition, cancer cells often spread to other organs, a process called **metastasis**. They can metastasize either by invading a nearby organ or by entering into the bloodstream or **lymphatic system** and traveling through the body to invade distant organs. Cancer cells can also make substances similar to hormones (called **growth factors**) which can stimulate other cancer or normal cells to grow (See Question 2).

A **tumor** is a mass of tissue formed by a new growth of cells. If a tumor stops growing by itself, and does not invade other tissues, it is considered **benign**. Examples include lipomas, which are soft, spongy, fatty tumors that form on the skin. Most tumors are **malignant**, which means they exhibit all the properties of cancer cells we've just mentioned.

2. What should I know about cancer cells?

One generalization is that most cancer cells have **mutations** in their **DNA**. DNA is the "brain" of the cell. However, the DNA is not scattered diffusely throughout the cell; it is organized into 46 discrete units called **chromosomes**. The chromosomes are located in the center of the cell, or **nucleus**. Each cell in the human body contains 46 chromosomes. These chromosomes are made up of thousands of smaller units called **genes**; each of these genes regulates a particular function. For example, certain genes control the color of your hair, others control how tall you grow, others control whether you produce insulin. If a gene is accidentally damaged, the change is called a **mutation**. It is not always clear as to what causes mutations. Some mutations are inherited, some may be due to diet, and others might be caused by exposure to environmental factors, such as radon, or cancer-causing chemicals (**carcinogens**). For example, tobacco in cigarette smoke contains hundreds of powerful carcinogens. Some mutations damage the gene or chromosome to the point where it causes the gene to stop working. This may result in the death of the cell, which is a relatively unusual cause of cancer. Cancer is usually due to the unregulated growth of cells, not their deaths.

Most mutations that cause cancer do so by causing the genes to work incorrectly. (Incidentally, many cancer cells

Lymphatic system

A vascular system that contains lymph nodes; cancer can spread through the lymphatic system.

Growth factors

Substances that stimulate cells to grow; drugs that help the bone marrow recover from the effects of chemotherapy (see also colony-stimulating factors).

Tumor

A mass of tissue formed by a new growth of cells.

Benign

Not cancerous; not life-threatening.

Malignant

Cancerous; cells that exhibit rapid, uncontrolled growth and can spread to other parts of the body.

Mutation

A damaged gene.

DNA (deoxyribonucleic acid)

The "brain" of a cell; chromosomes are composed of DNA.

Chromosomes

Strands of DNA and proteins in cell nucleus that carry units of heredity (genes).

THE BASICS

Nucleus

The center of the cell which contains the chromosomes.

Gene

Unit of heredity that regulates a particular function; located in a specific place on a chromosome.

Carcinogens

Cancer-causing substances.

Oncogene

A gene that, when mutated, can allow a cell to grow uncontrollably.

Tumor suppressor gene

A gene that can block cancer from developing.

Angiogenesis

The formation of new blood vessels that allows tumors to grow.

from different patients have similar mutations.) Many of these mutations that cause cancer occur in genes that govern how cells grow or how cells die. After a normal gene is mutated, it is called either an **oncogene** or **tumor suppressor gene**. Oncogenes are genes that normally help cells grow; when they are mutated, they cannot shut off, and the cells cannot stop growing. (Something like the gas pedal of a car being stuck in the "on" position.) Tumor suppressor genes are genes that normally make injured or mutated cells stop growing. If they become mutated, they usually stop functioning, thus allowing the abnormal cells to continue to grow without stopping (as if the brakes of a car stopped working).

We also know that growth factors can be important in the development of cancer. Growth factors are substances made by cancer cells or (sometimes) normal cells. Estrogen, for example, is a growth factor made in the ovaries which is required for breast and ovarian cells to function normally. However, it can also cause some types of breast cancer cells to grow and divide. Some growth factors made by cancer cells tell other cells to grow and divide. An example of this is vascular epithelial growth factor (VEGF), a growth factor made by cancer cells that stimulates growth of new blood vessels. This is one way that tumors encourage blood vessels to grow into them, which is another common characteristic of cancer: it often needs blood vessels to support its growth. New blood vessels rarely form in adults, except in certain circumstances such as wound healing or pregnancy. Blood vessels are necessary for a tumor to grow because they deliver oxygen and nutrients to the tumor. They can also sometimes serve as a "highway" for tumor cells to travel as they spread throughout the body. Formation of new blood vessels is sometimes called **angiogenesis** (angio = blood; genesis = new; angiogenesis = formation of new blood vessels) or **neovascularization** (neo = new; vascularization = development of blood vessels; neovascularization = development of new blood vessels). Another example of a growth factor is epidermal growth factor (EGF). (See Question 44)

3. *How do normal lungs function?*

Lungs are necessary for breathing—that is, bringing oxygen into the body and getting rid of carbon dioxide. Oxygen is necessary for cells to make energy. As this happens, the oxygen is used up and carbon dioxide is made. Carbon dioxide is a waste product, which needs to be removed from the body. This important oxygen-carbon dioxide exchange takes place in the lungs.

When we breathe in, or inhale, air travels through the main breathing tube called the **trachea**, which divides into two tubes (**main stem bronchi**) in the area near the heart. One tube goes to the right lung (right main stem bronchus) and the other to the left (left main stem bronchus). From there, the bronchi divide into smaller and smaller segments until they eventually become so tiny and thin that they are called alveoli. **Alveoli** are the millions of microscopic air sacs through which oxygen diffuses into red blood cells in the blood, where it is carried throughout the body. In exchange, carbon dioxide carried by the red blood cells from the body diffuses into the alveoli; it is then expelled out of the body through the airways when we exhale.

Notice that each lung is divided into sections called **lobes**. The right lung has three lobes, but the left lung has only two to make room for the heart. The heart assists in the vital process of breathing by pumping blood to and from the lungs (**Figure 1**).

Neovascularization

Formation of new blood vessels that allows tumors to grow.

THE BASICS

Trachea

Breathing tube (airway) leading from the larynx to the lungs.

Main stem bronchi

The two main breathing tubes (right main stem bronchus and left main stem bronchus) that branch off the trachea.

Alveoli

Tiny air sacs that compose the lungs.

Lobes

Clear anatomical divisions or extensions that can be determined without the use of a microscope (at the gross anatomy level). The right lung contains three lobes and the left contains two.

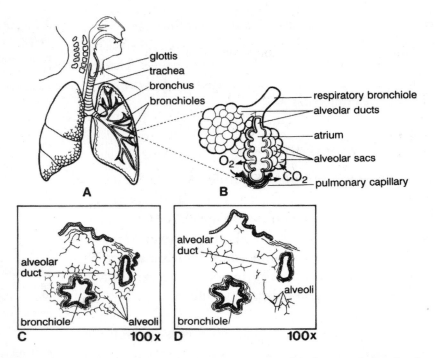

Figure 1 Internal structure of the lungs. A) Relationship of the lungs to the head and neck. B) External and internal appearance of a lung lobule, showing the atrium and alveolar sacs. C) Section of a lung, magnified 100 times. D) Section of a similar lung with emphysema. Note the decreased number of alveolar sacs and consequent diminishing in the gas exchange area of lung tissue.

Reprinted from Anderson PD and Spitzer VM: *Human Anatomy and Physiology Coloring Workbook and Study Guide,* Third Ed. Copyright © 2009, Jones and Bartlett Publishers, LLC

There are four major types of lung cancer: squamous cell carcinoma, adenocarcinoma, large cell carcinoma, and small cell carcinoma.

4. Are there different types of lung cancer?

There are four major types of lung cancer: **squamous cell carcinoma, adenocarcinoma, large cell carcinoma**, and **small cell carcinoma**. The primary difference between squamous cell, adenocarcinoma, and large cell carcinoma is how they look under the microscope. These three are sometimes collectively called **non-small cell lung cancer (NSCLC)**, to distinguish them from **small cell lung cancer (SCLC)**, or small cell carcinoma. In the United States, adenocarcinoma is the most common type of lung cancer, representing about 40% of all lung cancers. Sometimes, it is difficult to tell what type of NSCLC it is, in which case it may be called "poorly differentiated" or "NSCLC—not otherwise specified" (NSCLC-NOS).

Small cell lung cancer represents roughly 15%–20% of all lung cancers. It differs from the three types of non-small cell lung cancer in several important ways: it tends to be more rapidly growing, causes symptoms quicker, and spreads more rapidly. SCLC also tends to be more sensitive to **chemotherapy** and **radiation therapy** than NSCLC. For these reasons, patients with SCLC rarely undergo surgery. Instead, the standard treatment is chemotherapy, sometimes with radiation therapy (see Question 55).

Until very recently, squamous cell carcinoma, adeno-carcinoma, and large cell carcinoma were all treated the same way. However, more recent data suggests that some treatments may be more effective or safer in one subtype than another, such as bevacizumab or pemetrexed (see Question 44).

One sub-type of adenocarcinoma also bears mentioning: **bronchioloalveolar carcinoma (BAC)**. BAC is a rare form of lung cancer, representing only about 5% of all lung cancers; however, for unknown reasons, the number of patients developing BAC is rising. BAC is unique in that it tends to spread diffusely throughout the alveoli (see Question 3), unlike the more typical lung cancer cells, which tend to "stick together" and form solid, discrete masses. The cause of BAC is less clear than for other forms of lung cancer. It tends to occur in younger, nonsmoking women. Of all the types of lung cancer, it is the one that is most often found in patients who have never smoked, although it is also found in smokers. (For more information on BAC, see Question 63.)

THE BASICS

Squamous cell carcinoma

A type of non-small cell lung cancer.

Adenocarcinoma

A type of non-small cell lung cancer; a malignant tumor that arises from glandular tissue.

Large cell carcinoma

A type of non-small cell lung cancer.

Small cell carcinoma

A type of lung cancer that differs in appearance and behavior from non-small cell lung cancers (adenocarcinoma, squamous cell carcinoma, large cell carcinoma).

Non-small cell lung cancer (NSCLC)

A type of lung cancer that includes adeno-carcinoma, squamous cell carcinoma, and large cell carcinoma.

Small cell lung cancer (SCLC)

Refers to small cell carcinoma, as opposed to non-small cell lung cancers (adenocarcinoma, squamous cell carcinoma, large cell carcinoma).

5. What causes lung cancer?

Eighty-five to 90% of lung cancers are caused by carcinogens in tobacco that cause damage (mutations) to the DNA in lung cells. People are usually exposed to these carcinogens by directly inhaling them while smoking; however, people can sometimes develop lung cancer because they have inhaled large quantities of smoke from other smokers (**passive smoking**). Rarely, radon (a gas found underground) can also cause lung cancer. Exposure to asbestos, air pollution, and certain other environmental carcinogens can also cause lung cancer. When this occurs, it is usually a result of long-term, occupational exposure. (See Questions 98–99 for information on lung cancer risk, screening, and prevention.)

6. Who gets lung cancer? Is it common? Are the demographics changing?

Lung cancer is second only to prostate cancer in men and breast cancer in women in **incidence** (incidence is the number of new patients who develop a cancer in one year per 100,000 people). Unfortunately, it is a very deadly disease; despite being second in incidence, it is nevertheless the leading cause of cancer death among both men and women. Lung cancer is responsible for more cancer-related deaths than breast cancer, colon cancer, and prostate cancer combined. For unclear reasons, African-Americans have the highest incidence and death rates of lung cancer.

Lung cancer is most commonly found in current or former smokers, usually in their late 60s. The incidence of lung cancer has been on the rise since smoking became popular in the 1920s and 1930s, but it began to rise rapidly around 1960, when the effects of the "cigarette

Chemotherapy
The use of medicine to treat cancer; a "whole-body" or systemic treatment.

Radiation therapy
Treatment that uses high-dose x-rays or other high energy rays to kill cancer cells.

Bronchiolo-alveolar carcinoma (BAC)
A type of adenocarcinoma.

Passive smoking
Inhaling second-hand smoke.

Incidence
The number of new cases of a cancer (or any disease or event) in a defined population during a set period of time.

boom" during the World War II years became evident. The death rate for lung cancer in men peaked in the late 1980s; however, it continued to rise in women until roughly the year 2000, when it started to level off. Many people do not realize that lung cancer is the leading cancer killer of both men and women. Of note, although stopping smoking significantly decreases the risk of lung cancer, the risk never goes down to zero. Approximately 50% of all lung cancers occur in former smokers.

THE BASICS

PART TWO

Diagnosis and Staging

What are the most common symptoms of lung cancer?

Are there other symptoms associated with lung cancer?

How is lung cancer diagnosed?

What is staging and why is it important?

More . . .

7. What are the most common symptoms of lung cancer?

The symptoms of lung cancer depend upon its location. If a cancer occurs near the center of the chest, for example, it often presses on a major airway or blood vessel. In these cases, common symptoms include cough (including blood-tinged **sputum**) and shortness of breath. If the tumor blocks or obstructs a major airway, bacteria and secretions can back up behind the obstruction, resulting in a "post-obstructive" **pneumonia**.

Other structures near the center of the chest are sometimes affected by lung cancer. Rarely, the recurrent laryngeal nerve may be involved. The recurrent laryngeal nerve is a nerve that goes from the brain to the vocal cords. Because of the way humans develop as fetuses, this nerve does not make a direct path from the brain to the vocal cord, as one might expect. Instead, it travels down to the chest and then back up again, swinging by the major vessels leading in and out of the heart. If the tumor happens to press upon this nerve, hoarseness can result. Similarly, if the tumor happens to press on the **esophagus**, the "feeding tube" that leads from the mouth to the stomach, patients can experience problems with swallowing. If the tumor presses on one of the great vessels leading into the heart, such as the superior vena cava, the blood sometimes cannot flow easily into the heart. Instead, it backs up into the neck, shoulders, and arms (**superior vena cava syndrome**). In this case, patients can experience swelling of these areas.

If the tumor arises farther out in the lung near the chest wall, patients can experience pain. Indeed, this is often the only time patients experience pain from lung cancer

Sputum

Mucus and other secretions produced by the lungs.

Pneumonia

An infection of the lung.

Esophagus

The tube through which food travels from the mouth to the stomach.

Superior vena cava syndrome (SVCS)

A collection of symptoms that may include swelling in the neck, shoulders, and arms caused by a lung tumor pressing on the SVC, one of the large vessels leading into the heart.

because this is really the only area of the lung that has nerve endings. The middle of the lung and the area near the heart do not have many nerve endings, so tumors that arise in these areas rarely cause pain. This is one of the reasons why lung cancer can grow unnoticed for a long period of time: it is painless unless the chest wall is involved.

Tumors arising near the chest wall can also cause a **pleural effusion** (see Question 84). A pleural effusion is an accumulation of fluid between the outside of the lung and the inside of the chest wall. This fluid can cause pain, cough, and shortness of breath.

If the tumor occurs near the top of the lung, (**Pancoast tumor** or **superior sulcus tumor**) it may grow into some of the nerves leaving the spinal cord and traveling down through the armpit and into the arm. In this case, it can cause shoulder pain or weakness, or an unusual group of symptoms consisting of a droopy eyelid, dry eyes, and lack of sweating on the face.

If the tumor metastasizes, its symptoms will be related to the area of the body to which it has spread. For example, if the cancer spreads to the bone, it may cause pain in the back, hip, leg, or arm. If it spreads to the brain, it can cause headaches, nausea, or signs and symptoms similar to a stroke. These symptoms are not unique to metastatic lung cancer—any cancer that spreads to these organs will cause similar symptoms.

The most frequent symptoms of cancer, however, are fatigue, weakness, loss of appetite, and weight loss. These symptoms usually indicate that the cancer is advanced.

Pleural effusion

Accumulation of fluid between the outside of the lung and the inside of the chest wall.

Pancoast tumor (superior sulcus tumor)

A tumor occurring near the top of the lungs that may cause shoulder pain or weakness, or a group of symptoms including a droopy eyelid, dry eyes, and lack of sweating on the face.

The most frequent symptoms of cancer, however, are fatigue, weakness, loss of appetite, and weight loss. These symptoms usually indicate that the cancer is advanced.

8. Are there other symptoms associated with lung cancer?

Paraneoplastic symptoms

Symptoms that result from substances released by cancer cells and that occur at a site not directly involved with the tumor.

Electrolytes

Acids, bases, and salts essential for maintaining life; electrolyte abnormalities are imbalances of salts or chemicals in the blood.

Neuropathy

See **peripheral neuropathy**.

Clubbing

A condition that causes the nails on the fingers to bulge out; clubbing occurs with many different types of lung problems.

X-ray

High-energy radiation used to image the body.

Biopsy

Removal of tissue or fluid sample for microscopic examination.

Sometimes tumors can cause **paraneoplastic symptoms**. Paraneoplastic symptoms occur at a site not directly involved with the tumor. Presumably, the tumor must be making some type of hormone to affect these distant sites. Common paraneoplastic syndromes include **electrolyte** abnormalities (such as calcium and sodium imbalances), **neuropathy** (numbness and tingling of the hands and feet), and **clubbing** of the fingers. Clubbing can occur with many different types of lung problems (not only lung cancer). It is a word for the situation when the nails on the fingers bulge out somewhat. The cause of this effect is not known.

Patients with cancer are more susceptible to blood clots in the legs (deep veinous thromboses, or "DVTs"). This is a paraneoplastic syndrome that occurs when tumors generate substances that make the blood more prone to clotting.

9. How is lung cancer diagnosed?

The diagnosis of lung cancer frequently is made when a patient goes to his or her primary care physician complaining of cough, shortness of breath, and low-grade fevers. Because these symptoms are so common, the patient is often treated for a bronchitis or respiratory infection with antibiotics without taking a chest **x-ray**. If the symptoms do not go away, however, a chest x-ray is eventually obtained, revealing some type of mass in the chest. The x-ray is frequently followed by a chest CT scan to provide a better picture of the lungs and chest. This, in turn, often results in a **biopsy** (sampling of tissue), which is required for diagnosis of any type of cancer. (CT scan and biopsy are discussed further in Question 10.)

It is also not uncommon for lung cancer to be discovered accidentally on a chest x-ray or a CT scan taken for an unrelated condition. Currently, there is no approved screening test for lung cancer in **asymptomatic** (symptom-free) individuals who may be at risk for lung cancer (see Question 99).

10. Which tests are performed to diagnose lung cancer?

A computed tomography or CT scan (sometimes called a CAT scan) is the most helpful test for visualizing an abnormality in the lung. CT scans are a series of x-rays in which the body is "sliced up" like a pack of Lifesavers. Each one of the slices is then called up on a computer screen to give a cross-sectional image of the chest. A CT scan offers considerably more detail than a regular chest x-ray. To help the radiologist distinguish between blood vessels and tumors on CT scans, a dye called CT or IV contrast is sometimes injected into the vein to make the blood vessels more pronounced.

Once a suspicious abnormality is found on a CT scan, the patient needs a biopsy to obtain a diagnosis. There are several ways of doing this. These include:

- **Bronchoscopy.** A bronchoscopy is a procedure in which a lung doctor (**pulmonologist**) inserts a flexible tube called a **bronchoscope** through the nose down into the lungs. The bronchoscope, which has fiber-optic lighting inside, has several purposes. It can serve as a "periscope," allowing the pulmonologist to see into the airways. Additionally, needles can be inserted through the bronchoscope to obtain biopsies. The procedure is usually done as an out-patient under sedation.

Asymptomatic
Without symptoms.

Bronchoscopy
A procedure that involves inserting a flexible tube (bronchoscope) through the nose down into the lungs. Needles can be inserted through the bronchoscope to obtain biopsy samples.

Pulmonologist
A physician who specializes in the diagnosis and treatment of lung diseases.

Bronchoscope
See **bronchoscopy**.

DIAGNOSIS AND STAGING

15

Although bronchoscopy is a commonly used diagnostic test, it does have several disadvantages. First, the pulmonologist usually cannot get the tube into the distant areas of the lung—the airways near the chest wall are too small for the bronchoscope to get through. Therefore, the use of this test is limited to the larger bronchi, or airways. Second, if the cancer itself is not actually growing in the airway, it can be difficult for the pulmonologist to get a biopsy, because he or she cannot actually see the tumor.

Alternatives:

- **Transthoracic** or **percutaneous biopsy**. Specialized doctors, called **interventional radiologist**s, can sometimes insert a needle "from the outside in"—e.g. through the skin and chest wall into the tumor—in order to obtain tissue for a biopsy. This procedure usually does not require a hospital stay (it is an outpatient procedure) and is often done under a local anesthetic.
- Surgery. Sometimes, the abnormality seen on chest x-ray or CT scan cannot be easily biopsied by either a bronchoscopy or a transthoracic biopsy. In this case, patients may have to undergo a relatively minor surgical procedure under general anesthetic (and thus may require an overnight stay in the hospital). The surgeon can do several different procedures to make the diagnosis. These include:
- **Mediastinoscopy**. This procedure involves making a small incision above the collarbone or between the spaces of the first and second or second and third ribs. The surgeon then inserts a special tube through this incision into the **mediastinum**. Again, this tube has two functions: it allows the surgeon to see the **lymph nodes** near the heart, and it also allows the surgeon

Transthoracic (percutaneous) biopsy

A biopsy obtained by inserting a needle through the skin and chest wall into the tumor.

Interventional radiologist

A radiologist who uses x-rays and other imaging techniques to perform minimally invasive medical procedures.

Mediastinoscopy

A surgical procedure by which lymph nodes can be removed for microscopic examination.

Mediastinum

Area between the lungs.

Lymph node

Small collections of white blood cells scattered throughout the body.

to biopsy them. A mediastinoscopy is sometimes done not only to make the diagnosis of cancer, but also to help "stage" the patient (see Question 13).

- **Mini-thoracotomy** or **video-assisted thoracoscopic surgery (VATS)**. Both of these procedures involve making an incision someplace on the outside of the chest and inserting a tube into the space between the chest wall and the lung. This allows a surgeon to see the outside of the lung and to biopsy any suspicious areas.

11. How will I learn about the results of my biopsy? What information will be in the pathology report, and what will it mean for me?

It typically takes two to three days before the biopsy results become available. We strongly suggest that you schedule an appointment with your doctor to receive the results and discuss your **prognosis** and treatment options. There is nothing worse than getting bad news over the phone, when the doctor may not have much time to talk to you.

A specialized doctor called a **pathologist** looks at the biopsy samples under the microscope. He or she tries to answer the following critical questions:

- Is it cancer? The pathologist determines this by judging how "normal" the cells look. Part of the definition of cancer is that cells look very abnormal and no longer look or function like the type of cells they are supposed to be. The question as to whether something is cancerous is not always black or white. Typically, normal cells from different parts of our body look very different microscopically and are easy to tell

Mini-thoracotomy
A type of minimally invasive chest surgery.

Video-assisted thoracoscopic surgery (VATS)
A type of minimally invasive chest surgery.

It typically takes two to three days before the biopsy results become available.

Prognosis
Predicted outcome; likelihood of survival.

Pathologist
A physician trained to examine and evaluate cells and tissue.

DIAGNOSIS AND STAGING

apart—blood cells look very different from muscle cells, for example. In many tumors, however, the cells are so wildly abnormal looking that one cannot tell where they originated from or from what part of the body they were taken, in which case they are called "poorly differentiated." In other cases the cells may look "abnormal" and in others "somewhat abnormal." Pathologists use the term "**differentiation**" to describe the degree of abnormality of the appearance of the cells. A "well differentiated" adenocarcinoma, for example, looks somewhat like normal lung cells. Generally speaking, the more differentiated a cancer looks, the better.

Differentiation

A term used to describe the degree to which tumor tissue resembles normal tissue.

- If it is cancer, what kind is it? As discussed in Question 4, there are different types of lung cancer. Although the pathologist typically will call it one of the four major types (adenocarcinoma, squamous cell carcinoma, large cell carcinoma, or small cell carcinoma) based on its appearance microscopically, the most important distinction is whether or not it is small cell lung cancer.

Pathologists classify tumors into different **histological** types based upon the characteristics or patterns some tumors make. For example, adenocarcinomas often look like glands; large cell carcinomas contain—you guessed it—large cancer cells; and small cell cancers contain small cancer cells. As it turns out, many cancers that start in different parts of the body can also look glandular. For example, breast cancer, colon cancer, and prostate cancers are also adenocarcinomas. Sometimes, they are hard to tell apart.

Histology/ Histological

Tissue type; assessment of cellular feautres by microscopic evaluation.

- If it is cancer, where did it come from? If a tumor starts in the lung, it is called lung cancer. However, other cancers commonly spread to the lungs. If a tumor starts elsewhere in the body, say, the breast, and spreads to the lung, it is still called breast cancer. If a lung cancer spreads to the liver, for example, it is still called lung cancer. This is because in general, cancers typically behave like the cancer where it came from—breast cancer that has spread or metastasized to the lung still tends to respond to breast cancer chemotherapy better than lung cancer chemotherapy, and tends to grow and behave similarly to breast cancer elsewhere in the body.

Sometimes, the cancer may look so very abnormal, the pathologist cannot tell where it came from, or cannot distinguish between the different types of lung cancer, in which case he or she may call it a "poorly differentiated cancer." Usually, however, the pathologist is able to distinguish a non-small cell lung cancer from small-cell lung cancer. Don't worry if the pathologist cannot differentiate between adenocarcinoma, squamous cell carcinoma, or large cell carcinoma—in the past, we have generally treated all non-small cell carcinomas the same. More recently, however, there is data indicating that patients with squamous cell carcinoma may not respond as well to a type of chemotherapy called pemetrexed, or Alimta; although at the time of this writing that has not been definitively proven. Also, patients with squamous cell carcinoma are more likely to have side effects from bevacizumab (Avastin), so bevacizumab is rarely given to these patients.

12. What are lymph nodes?

Lymph nodes are small collections of white blood cells scattered throughout the body. White blood cells not only flow through the bloodstream, they also flow through a second type of vascular system in our bodies called the lymphatic system. Unlike the other organs in our body, of which everyone has the same number (e.g., we all have two lungs, one liver, one heart), there are hundreds of different lymph nodes scattered throughout the body, and everyone has a slightly different number of them.

Lymph nodes are important because sometimes cancer can spread through the lymphatic system. If the lymph nodes that your surgeon removes contain cancer, this implies that since your lung cancer got that far, it may also have passed through the lymph nodes and spread elsewhere in your body.

13. What is staging, and why is it important?

Staging

Determining where the cancer is and how far cancer has spread.

Staging a tumor involves determining where the tumor is, its size, and how far a cancer has spread. This is useful for several reasons:

- It allows physicians to have a common "language" in describing a patient's tumor. Thus, when a surgeon tells an oncologist that a patient has Stage IIIA lung cancer, the oncologist immediately has some idea as to the extent of the patient's disease.

- It is an important prognostic indicator. Patients with Stage I disease, for example, typically do much better than do patients with Stage IV disease.

  It is very useful for determining therapy. The type of treatment that is recommended—surgery, radiotherapy, chemotherapy, or any combination of these—will depend upon the extent of the disease and how far it has spread.

14. What are the staging guidelines for NSCLC?

The staging of cancer is classically dependent upon three criteria: the size and location of the tumor (T or tumor status); whether any lymph nodes are involved (N or nodal status); and whether the cancer has spread further than the lymph nodes (M or metastatic status). These three criteria (T, N, and M) are further subdivided. For example, if no lymph nodes contain tumor, this is called N0; if the local, (or **hilar**), lymph nodes contain tumor, this is called N1; and if the lymph nodes between the lung and the heart, (the **mediastinal lymph nodes**), contain tumor, this is typically called N2. N3 disease involves the lymph nodes in the other side of the chest, or in the area above the collar bone.

Oncologists use a complicated system, based upon the TNM staging, to determine the overall stage. A simplified summary of the current (2008) staging system is provided in **Table 1**. However, it should be noted that the staging system may change slightly in 2009.

15. What are the staging guidelines for small cell lung cancer (SCLC)?

Because SCLC tends to metastasize early, oncologists typically do not go into the formal "TNM" staging classification noted above. Instead, they typically divide SCLC into "limited stage" or "extensive stage" disease, in which limited stage is defined as cancer confined to one side of the chest, and extensive stage is defined as cancer that has spread outside the side of the chest from which it arose.

Hilar lymph nodes

Lymph nodes located in the region where the bronchus meets the lung.

Mediastinal lymph nodes

Lymph nodes located in the mediastinum, the area between the lungs.

Table 1 Lung cancer staging based upon the TNM staging criteria

Stage I	Tumors that are small and do not have any lymph node involvement
Stage II	Tumors that have spread to the local (hilar) lymph nodes, OR tumors abutting the chest wall without lymph node involvement
Stage III	Tumors that are "locally advanced" but do not appear to have metastasized to distant organs
Stage IIIA	Tumors that are large and bulky but are still surgically resectable (i.e., the surgeon is technically able to take the tumor out), OR tumors that have spread to the mediastinal lymph nodes
Stage IIIB	Tumors that have not yet metastasized, but that are too large to resect or that are located such that the surgeon would be unable to resect them safely. Typical examples are tumors that have invaded the heart, one of the large blood vessels leading into or out of the heart, or one of the major airways. Also, patients with pleural effusion (see Question 84) and N3 lymph node (see Question 14) involvement are classified as having Stage IIIB disease.
Stage IV	Tumors that have spread to other organs (metastatic)

16. What are the common metastatic sites for lung cancer?

The most common metastatic sites for both non-small cell and small cell lung cancer are elsewhere in the lungs, the liver, the adrenal glands, the bones, and the brain.

17. Which tests and procedures are used to detect whether my lung cancer has spread beyond my chest?

Your oncologist may order a series of tests to determine whether the cancer has spread to one of the sites mentioned above. These might include a **bone scan** (an imaging test in which a radionuclear substance is injected into the veins and taken up by cancer cells, if any, in the bones), a head or abdominal **CT scan**, or a **PET scan**. PET (positron emission tomography) is a nuclear medicine scan that measures metabolism, or how quickly cells break down nutrients for energy. Because cancer cells grow faster than normal cells, they presumably need more energy than normal cells. Since cancer cells get their energy from sugar, or glucose, they are more likely to use more glucose than normal cells, a difference that can be picked up on a PET scan. PET scans are most often used at the time of diagnosis to help stage a patient. In particular, it is often used to help the surgeon to decide which lymph nodes may have cancer and therefore should be biopsied.

PET scans are not perfect, however. White blood cells also use a lot of glucose. Thus, any infection or irritation ("inflammation") may also be positive on PET scan (a "false positive"). In addition, broncheoalveolar cancers are sometimes so slow growing that they do not use a lot of glucose and thus can be falsely negative on PET scan. Finally, our brains use so much glucose that it is difficult to see a cancer or tumor in the brain on PET scan.

Bone scan

An imaging test in which a radionuclear substance is injected into the veins and taken up by the bones in areas of potential metastatic disease.

CT scan (computed tomography)

Computerized series of x-rays that create a detailed cross-sectional image of the body.

PET scan (positron emission tomography)

A nuclear medicine imaging test that measures metabolism; can differentiate between healthy and abnormal tissue.

PART THREE

I've Just Been Diagnosed with Lung Cancer— Now What?

Who treats lung cancer? What is multidisciplinary care?

Should I get a second opinion?

How can I relate best to my doctor? What can I do to make my medical visits as productive as possible?

More . . .

18. Who treats lung cancer? What is multidisciplinary care?

You likely will see more than one specialist for your lung cancer care, including medical oncologists, thoracic surgeons, radiation oncologists, and pulmonologists.

Lung cancer is a complex disease, and its treatment frequently involves some combination of surgery, chemotherapy and radiation. (see Questions 34, 39, and 46) You likely will see more than one specialist for your lung cancer care, including medical oncologists, thoracic surgeons, radiation oncologists, and pulmonologists. Ideally, these lung cancer doctors work together in a multidisciplinary clinic or other setting where they can easily consult with each other and together about your treatment options. This multidisciplinary approach not only offers you high-quality care but also has practical advantages that may include fewer trips to the doctor, less time from diagnosis to start of treatment, and more efficient coordination of the logistics involving treatment. Multidisciplinary care is commonly offered in cancer centers and in larger treatment centers such as university hospitals, but it is beginning to be implemented in some community hospitals as well.

Each lung cancer specialist you see is a member of your treatment team, but one doctor (usually the medical oncologist) will have primary responsibility for managing and directing your care.

Medical oncologist

A physician who performs comprehensive management of cancer patients throughout all phases of care; specializes in treating cancer with medicine.

There are also a number of other doctors, along with support staff, who will be involved in your care. It is helpful to understand what each of these healthcare professionals does, and what role he or she plays in your care.

- **Medical oncologist**: a physician who performs comprehensive management of cancer patients throughout all phases of care. Medical oncologists specialize in treating cancer with medicine, using **systemic** treatments such as chemotherapy.

- **Thoracic surgeon**: a physician who specializes in performing chest surgery. A thoracic surgeon may have performed the tumor biopsy that resulted in your lung cancer diagnosis. Some thoracic surgeons have received additional training in cancer surgery and are considered surgical oncologists.

- **Radiation oncologist**: a physician who specializes in treating cancer with radiation.

- **Pulmonologist**: a physician who specializes in the diagnosis and treatment of lung diseases. A pulmonologist may have diagnosed your lung cancer. You may also see a pulmonologist if you have ongoing respiratory issues related to your lung cancer, or underlying conditions such as bronchitis, emphysema, or **chronic obstructive pulmonary disease** (COPD).

Other specialists or support staff:

- **Pathologist**: a physician trained to examine and evaluate cells and tissue under the microscope. The pathologist evaluates your biopsy tissue and furnishes a biopsy report to your oncologist or surgeon.

- **Oncology nurse**: a specialized nurse trained to provide care to cancer patients, including administering chemotherapy and monitoring side effects.

- Psychiatrist: a physician who specializes in treating people for depression, anxiety, and other psychological illness. Psychiatrists provide psychotherapy and can also prescribe medication.

- Psychologist: a person trained in psychology who can provide psychotherapy to help patients and their families better cope with their disease.

Systemic
Affecting the entire body.

Thoracic surgeon
A surgeon who specializes in performing chest surgery.

Radiation oncologist
A physician who specializes in treating cancer with radiation.

Pulmonologist
A physician who specializes in the diagnosis and treatment of lung diseases.

Chronic obstructive pulmonary disease (COPD)
Chronic bronchitis or emphysema.

Pathologist
A physician trained to examine and evaluate cells and tissues.

Oncology nurse
A specialized nurse trained to provide care to cancer patients.

Oncology social worker

A social worker trained to provide counseling and practical assistance to cancer patients.

Rehabilitation specialist

A person trained to help patients recover from physical changes brought about by cancer or cancer treatment.

Palliative care specialist

A physician trained in pain management.

One of your primary responsibilities as a lung cancer patient is to be sure that you are getting the best care possible, starting with your choice of doctors.

- **Oncology social worker**: a social worker trained to provide counseling and practical assistance to cancer patients. Social workers can help you locate services such as transportation, support groups, and home care. They can also provide assistance with insurance and financial issues.

- **Rehabilitation specialist**: a person trained to help patients recover from physical changes brought about by cancer or cancer treatment. Respiratory therapists help lung cancer patients to maximize their breathing capacity and learn to cope with breathlessness. Physical therapists can help patients recover range of motion and strength following lung cancer surgery.

- Nutritionist or dietician: a person trained to provide nutritional or dietary counseling. Lung cancer patients may experience weight loss as a result of their cancer or its treatment (see Question 86). Treatment side effects, such as nausea from chemotherapy or heartburn from radiation, can negatively affect appetite. Nutritional or dietary counseling services can help patients to increase appetite and gain weight.

- **Palliative care specialist**: a physician trained in managing cancer pain and other symptoms of cancer.

19. How do I find the best doctors to treat my lung cancer? Does the hospital make any difference in my care?

One of your primary responsibilities as a lung cancer patient is to be sure that you are getting the best care possible, starting with your choice of doctors. Although it is often difficult for patients to assess the quality of doctors and treatment centers, there are resources you can turn to, and questions you can ask, to help you decide on the right doctor for you.

The first step in finding a doctor or treatment center is to get a recommendation from a reliable source. Your primary care physician, or another doctor, can refer you to the best lung cancer specialists in your area. Other lung cancer patients are also good sources. If you cannot get a recommendation for a specific lung cancer specialist, you can contact the nearest cancer center or university hospital and ask for the names of their oncologists who specialize in lung cancer. The leading cancer centers are identified by the National Cancer Institute as NCI-designated cancer centers. The American College of Surgeons' Commission on Cancer also identifies hospitals with strong cancer programs. (For further information on these resources, and on others that will help you to locate doctors and cancer treatment centers, see Appendix A.)

After you have the name of a doctor, you need to evaluate whether this person is a quality physician. Equally important, you need to decide whether you are comfortable with this person and whether the two of you will be able to communicate well with each other as you face the difficult decisions that lie ahead.

Some things to consider:

- *Experience or expertise in lung cancer.* It is extremely important to find out whether a physician has extensive experience with lung cancer patients. Oncologists treat patients with all types of cancers, but ideally you want to find an oncologist who specializes in lung cancer. This type of oncologist is referred to as a thoracic (or lung) oncologist and may be found at major cancer centers. Similarly, if you are seeking a surgeon you want to find a thoracic surgeon who specializes in lung cancer surgery, and not a cardiac surgeon who specializes in heart surgery or a general surgeon who performs all types of surgeries. Studies have shown that the complication rate is lower for lung cancer surgery when the surgery is performed by a thoracic surgeon. You should ask any prospective oncologist or surgeon what percentage of his or her practice is lung cancer patients.

- *Hospital affiliation.* It is important to consider your doctor's hospital affiliation. Cancer centers and university hospitals conduct research and provide access to the newest treatments and to **clinical trials** (see Questions 59 and 60). Patients are more likely to receive multidisciplinary care in these institutions and benefit from the collective expertise of multiple specialists. Patients who undergo surgery for lung cancer at hospitals that perform a large volume of lung surgery are likely to survive longer and have fewer complications than patients who have similar surgery at hospitals with a low volume of lung cancer procedures.

Clinical trials

Research studies involving people.

You should be aware that cancer centers and university hospitals tend to be larger than community hospitals and often have fellows (doctors who are learning to be oncologists), residents (doctors in training) or medical students who see patients with the medical oncologist; however, even in these "teaching hospitals" your care will be directed by the medical oncologist, who should be seeing you at every visit with the fellow or resident. This may seem confusing, especially at the beginning, but most people get used to these differences. Hospital affiliation should be a major factor in deciding who your physician will be.

- *Credentials.* Basic professional information for licensed U.S. physicians is available through the American Medical Association's Physician Select web site, *www.ama-assn.org/aps/amahg.htm*. Each listing offers information on the physician's medical school, residency and fellowship training, board certification, and office location. Board certification ensures expertise in a specified area, such as medical oncology, radiation oncology, or thoracic surgery. Residency or fellowship training at a major cancer center can be a plus.

Other factors to consider:

- *Is the doctor covered by your insurance plan?* Financial constraints are a reality, and insurance is a limiting factor when selecting a doctor. There may be overriding reasons for consulting a specialist (or getting a second opinion) outside an insurance plan, but your primary lung cancer doctor needs to be covered by your policy unless cost is not an issue for you. Most insurances will allow you to get a second opinion outside your system, although they may not allow you to stay with that doctor.

- *Distance.* Certain types of treatment (e.g., chemotherapy and radiation) require multiple trips to the doctor or hospital. For some people, distance from the doctor will be a significant issue. Ask the hospital social worker about transportation alternatives or possibilities for inexpensive lodging. If you really like the doctor but are worried about the distance you will have to travel, particularly if you are feeling tired or sick, ask whether the oncologist and your primary doctor would be willing to work together. Some doctors feel very comfortable with this type of arrangement, while others do not.

- *Alternative medicine.* If you are interested in alternative medicine, you should address this issue during your first visit. It is crucial that both you and your doctor

It typically takes two to three days before the biopsy results become available.

are comfortable discussing alternative medicine issues and that you are open with your doctor about any use of alternative medicine (see Questions 61).

Trust and rapport are central to a strong doctor—patient relationship and should be given full consideration.

Because you are choosing a doctor who will be helping you to face life and death issues, the doctor's bedside manner, and your personal connection with him or her, are things to consider seriously. Trust and rapport are central to a strong doctor—patient relationship and should be given full consideration. Questions to ask yourself are:

- Does the doctor communicate in a clear and understandable manner? Is he or she willing to answer my questions? Is he or she a good listener, or did he or she appear rushed?
- Does the doctor appear knowledgeable? Does the doctor inspire confidence?
- Does the doctor seem compassionate, caring, trustworthy?
- Did the doctor ask about me and my family—is he or she looking beyond my lung cancer?

After your appointment or consultation, you should have a positive feeling that you and your doctor can work together as partners. If you are not comfortable with the first doctor you visit, you should not hesitate to look for another one.

On the other hand, you should remember that doctors are people, too. Although every patient would like to have a doctor who is a world-class, internationally-known researcher with lots of time to spend with individual patients and has a wonderful bedside manner, this isn't always going to be possible. The bottom line is that you need to feel comfortable that your doctor knows what he or she is doing, is interested in you as an individual, and is willing to talk to you and answer your questions.

Finally, don't "kill the messenger." Sometimes it is hard to separate the bad news from the person who has to give it. Just as it is not easy being on the receiving end of bad news, it is not easy being on the delivering end. Don't let your emotions about the diagnosis unfairly color your objective opinion of your doctor.

20. Should I get a second opinion?

The quality of your medical care is a critical factor in determining your chances for survival. A second opinion is an effective way to be sure you are getting the best possible care and, at the same time, to gain peace of mind that you have explored all of your options.

There are certain cases when a second opinion is particularly important:

- If you have been told that you are not a candidate for surgery but have reason to think you might be, you should seek another opinion from a thoracic surgeon. Surgery offers the best chance for a cure from lung cancer, and thoughts about who is a surgical candidate are changing. Thoracic surgeons who specialize in resecting lung cancers may be able to operate on some patients a general surgeon is not. Some patients become candidates for surgery after chemotherapy and/or radiation are used to shrink their tumors.

- If your doctor tells you that there is no treatment available for you, don't give up. It is rarely the case that there are no treatment options. A second opinion provides a different perspective and may bring additional choices for treatment.

A second opinion is an effective way to be sure you are getting the best possible care and, at the same time, to gain peace of mind that you have explored all of your options.

- If your doctor is associated with a small community hospital, it is a good idea to get a second opinion at a major cancer center or university hospital where research is performed, where the doctors may be more aware of the newest treatments, and where there may be additional clinical trial options for you.

- If you are uncomfortable with your doctor or have doubts about her recommendations for your care, you should look for another doctor. It is impossible to have a good doctor–patient relationship if you do not have confidence and trust in your doctor.

- If there is a question about your diagnosis (whether you have cancer, where it came from, or your tumor type), you should get a second pathology opinion (see Question 21). Errors in pathology are unusual but can occur. Your prognosis and treatment plan are determined by your pathological diagnosis, the diagnosis made by a pathologist after looking at your biopsy under a microscope. It is essential that your diagnosis is accurate.

Even when there is no compelling dilemma to resolve, a second opinion is still advisable. It can offer new options, confirm recommendations, or bring to light substandard care. If you get a conflicting second opinion, you can resolve issues by seeking a third opinion or by asking your primary care doctor (or another doctor) for guidance. Before seeking a second opinion, however, you should consider the potential downsides. The process of obtaining a second opinion can be emotionally draining, and will consume time and energy that you may not have. It can create confusion and delay treatment. You need to decide whether these negatives are offset by the potential long-term benefits of getting a second opinion.

Some patients worry that they will offend their doctor if they seek a second opinion. Keep in mind that you are entitled to seek a second opinion. Doctors are professionals who understand that patients will be seeking additional opinions or consultations. If you sense that your doctor is threatened by your intention to get a second opinion, then you might consider that to be further reason to pursue another perspective.

Unless you require emergency care, *you should try to get a second opinion before starting treatment.* This cannot be stressed enough. Once you have started treatment, it will be very difficult to switch to something else. Your doctor can advise you on how long you can afford to delay treatment. In the majority of cases, a few weeks won't make a difference to your health, and it makes sense to consider all options before making any treatment decision. There are also occasions after you have begun treatment when you may want to seek a second opinion; for example, if your disease is progressing and you are re-evaluating your treatment plan.

To make sure you get an independent assessment, it is a good idea to seek a second opinion from a doctor associated with a different institution than your original doctor. Many insurance companies will pay for second opinions, but it may be worth paying out of pocket for a second opinion from a particularly well-qualified specialist, even if he or she is outside your plan.

21. How do I go about getting a second opinion?

Arranging for a second opinion involves some logistics. You need to gather your medical records—including all reports and scans—to bring with you for a second opinion visit. We suggest hand-carrying them because outside records have a very bad habit of getting delayed (or lost) in the mail. *Remember—if you have had x-rays or scans done in more than one place, you will need to go to each place to get them.* The most important scans are your most recent CT scans and PET scan. Ask the person who gives them to you to double check to make sure they are in the package or on the disc. This cannot be overemphasized! Nothing is more frustrating than to get to the new doctor's office and find out the most recent scans are not there, despite the fact you were assured they would be.

You also will need to get your pathology slides. A second pathology opinion is typically part of the second-opinion process. If you are satisfied with your care but would just like to confirm your pathology, this can be done easily without an office visit. The Armed Forces Institute of Pathology is considered a leading pathology lab for second opinions. You can contact the AFIP by phone at 202-782-1630, or via their web site at *www.afip.org.*

22. How can I relate best to my doctor? What can I do to make my medical visits as productive as possible?

The doctor–patient relationship lies at the heart of patient care. This relationship will guide and support you throughout the course of your lung cancer. It is your job, and your doctor's, to nurture this relationship and to work toward a partnership based on mutual trust and respect. Although difficulties between doctor and patient may occur at times, just as they do in any relationship, these problems will be minimized if good communication is maintained. Remember that your doctor is not a mind reader. It is your responsibility to be open and honest and to bring up any concerns, needs or preferences you may have. It is especially important that you feel comfortable discussing sensitive issues such as your use of alternative medicine treatments, your lifestyle (smoking, drinking, drugs), end-of-life issues, and sexual concerns. Keep in mind that conversations between doctor and patient are confidential (your family does not need to know if you don't want them to) and that the more your doctor knows about issues that may impact your health, the better care you will receive.

It is your responsibility to be open and honest and to bring up any concerns, needs or preferences you may have.

At your first visit you should address the issues of how much information you want from your doctor and how involved you would like to be in the decisions that are made about your care. Some patients want to know everything about their condition, and they want to make all the decisions themselves. Some patients find too much information anxiety-provoking. These patients would prefer to hear less information (or only the good news) and are more comfortable allowing their doctor to make all the decisions. Many patients fall somewhere in between. Whatever your preferences may be, and they may change over time, you need to communicate them to your doctor. If you feel that your doctor is not responsive to your needs, or if you have other concerns regarding your relationship, you should bring them up before they reach a crisis stage. If you and your doctor cannot resolve disagreements in a productive and satisfactory manner, you should look for another doctor.

It is also important to discuss with your doctor how much you do or do not want your family involved. If you do not want your doctor discussing your case with family members without you present, tell your doctor. Most doctors will ask you to sign a "release of information" form, giving them permission to talk to whoever you designate, before they will talk to a friend or family member when you are not around.

Think about what you are going to say to your doctor ahead of time. Remember, he or she has a certain amount of time to spend with you, so before your appointment consider which concerns are most pressing and write them down in order of importance. This tactic will help you focus and make the most effective use of the limited time you have with your doctor. Too often, patients spend their time with the doctor trying to remember if the pain started on Monday, when Aunt Ellie was visiting for dinner, or on Tuesday afternoon, when they went out shopping, or Tuesday morning before breakfast or maybe Wednesday when Aunt Ellie came back to pick up the casserole dish she forgot. If you choose to review events in great detail, you risk running out of the time that your doctor has for addressing more important issues.

If you have symptoms to report, describe them clearly and concisely. Be prepared to answer your doctor's questions, such as when the symptoms started, how often they occur, and how long they last. In most instances, you do not have to be exact; saying "early last week" or "about 2 months ago" will suffice. Don't be afraid to mention the emotional and social issues that are affecting you, in addition to any physical problems you have.

Always bring someone with you to your appointment. It is impossible to remember all that is said during an office visit, and emotions can cloud what a patient hears. It helps to have someone else along who can write down what the doctor says. Tape recording your conversations are another very helpful way of remembering exactly what transpired. As long as you tell the doctor what you are doing, most physicians have no problem with this. It is important that you understand everything that your doctor tells you. If something is unclear, say so, and ask questions until you are satisfied that you understand completely.

Many oncologists have an oncology nurse or nurse practitioner with whom they work closely. *Get this person's name and number!* He or she can answer a lot of questions the doctor may not have time for, particularly between visits, and is often your "patient advocate" with your doctor. In many cases, he or she will be the "go between" you and your doctor, particularly between visits when problems or questions come up.

Be sure that all necessary tests are completed prior to your visit and that you have all the information you need. This includes having the required referrals, if any, and a current list of the prescription and nonprescription drugs you are taking. (It is very helpful to *bring the actual pill bottles along with EACH visit).* Bring a notebook or binder that contains your medical information and paperwork to each appointment. If you can present your doctor with the information she needs to care for you in an efficient and clear manner, you will go a long way toward increasing the quality of your relationship with your doctor and, ultimately, the quality of your care.

PART FOUR

Coping with Your Diagnosis

What is my prognosis? Can I survive lung cancer?

How do I manage my emotions? Should I seek professional counseling? What types of psychosocial support are available to me?

How do I regain control of my life after my lung cancer diagnosis? How do I get past the emotional impact and move forward?

More . . .

23. What is my prognosis? Can I survive lung cancer?

It is natural to worry about what a lung cancer diagnosis will mean for you and your family and to wonder whether you will die from your cancer. Most patients want to know their prognosis so that they can plan for the future and prepare for what lies ahead. Your prognosis is a prediction of how well you will do and how long you will live. It is influenced by many factors, including the type of lung cancer you have, how far your cancer has spread, how aggressive your tumor is, your age, and your general health. The treatment you receive may affect your prognosis, and your prognosis may change over time. The best person to discuss your prognosis with is your doctor.

To arrive at your prognosis, your doctor will take into consideration the lung cancer statistics, his or her experience with other lung cancer patients, and what he or she knows about your individual case.

To arrive at your prognosis, your doctor will take into consideration the lung cancer statistics, his or her experience with other lung cancer patients, and what he or she knows about your individual case. It is important to remember that your prognosis is only an educated guess and that it is impossible for anyone, even your doctor, to predict your future with certainty.

You may become familiar with the survival statistics for lung cancer through discussions with your doctor or from other sources. For lung cancer patients, survival rates are not encouraging, and it can be overwhelming to learn about them. It is helpful to understand why these statistics may not be accurate for you. Survival statistics, like those compiled by the American Cancer Society, usually measure the 5-year survival of a group of patients with similar characteristics. They are "averages" and do not represent the prognosis for any given individual. Your unique characteristics will cause your prognosis to differ from the "average" lung cancer patient. You should also be aware that the survival statistics reflect the outcomes of patients who were treated with older therapies. They don't take into account the newer, more effective treatments that are available today, or the promising treatments that will be available in the near future.

Although it makes sense to plan for every eventuality when you are facing a potentially deadly disease, you should not allow statistics or a bleak prediction by your doctor to dictate your future. There are patients who have survived every stage of lung cancer and patients who have outlived their doctors' predictions. Your prognosis provides a perspective, but it is not etched in stone. Try to focus your thoughts on the tens of thousands of people who have survived lung cancer. There is no reason why you can't be one of them.

Having said all that, however, while it is good to "hope for the best," you should also "prepare for the worst." Now is a good time to assess your personal, financial, and legal affairs (see Questions 29 and 97). Working on these issues while you are undergoing treatment in no way means you are "giving up." It may, however, relieve you of other worries down the road.

EMOTIONAL ASPECTS

24. How do I manage my emotions? Should I seek professional counseling? What types of psychosocial support are available to me?

A lung cancer diagnosis brings with it a tidal wave of emotions and a sense of uncertainty about the future.

Feelings of shock, denial, anger, fear, helplessness, sadness, and anxiety are all normal responses to a life-threatening crisis. You likely will experience a range of emotions that will fluctuate from moment to moment and vary over the course of your disease. It is important to remember that there is no right or wrong way to feel and that it can take time to learn to cope with your emotions. You may hear from others that you can influence your chances for survival through positive thinking and an upbeat attitude. Although this approach may be helpful to you, you should not worry that feelings of anger or sadness will cause your tumor to grow faster—this is a common worry among cancer patients, but there is no evidence that it occurs. Expressing your emotions, both positive and negative, can be an effective way to relieve stress. You should feel comfortable using whatever coping mechanisms work for you and not be concerned about being a "perfect" cancer patient.

One method of coping that works well for many cancer patients is to reach out to others for emotional support. Spending time with family, friends, neighbors, and members of your religious community may help to reduce the sense of isolation brought on by your cancer diagnosis. In particular, connecting with other lung cancer survivors can be heartening and inspiring. People who are facing similar challenges share common concerns, experiences, and hopes for the future. The National Lung Cancer Partnership (*www.NationalLungCancerPartnership.org*) provides educational materials and resources for those dealing with a diagnosis of lung cancer. The Lung Cancer Alliance (LCA) provides a phone buddy program that will pair you with someone who has a similar type and stage of lung cancer. LCA also maintains a geographic listing of in-person lung cancer support groups. Support groups are not for everyone, but if you are looking for a community of people who will know exactly how you feel and can offer emotional support and practical information, a lung cancer support group will likely meet your needs. If no group is available in your area or if you are reticent to participate in an in-person group, you might consider joining an online support group (also called a discussion list or a mailing list). The Association for Cancer Online Resources (ACOR) maintains four lung cancer lists: a general list (LUNG-ONC), and specific lists for small cell lung cancer (LUNG-SCLC), non-small cell lung cancer (LUNG-NSCLC), and bronchioloalveolar carcinoma (LUNG-BAC). Online support groups are especially valuable for patients who are physically unable to attend in-person groups but who wish to participate in a lung cancer community. (See Question 100 for information about locating lung cancer support groups.)

If you find that your distress persists and that you are having ongoing difficulty managing your emotions, you may want to seek mental health, social work, or pastoral counseling. Your doctor can refer you to a psychiatrist or psychologist who can evaluate your symptoms and provide therapy to help relieve your distress. Clinical social workers can also provide counseling and can alert you to other sources of support. Mental health professionals can teach you coping strategies such as relaxation techniques and guided imagery. Your religion can provide comfort at this time, and you may want to approach your clergy about spiritual counseling.

If you find that your distress persists and that you are having ongoing difficulty managing your emotions, you may want to seek mental health, social work, or pastoral counseling.

25. How do I regain control of my life after my lung cancer diagnosis? How do I get past the emotional impact and move forward?

A lung cancer diagnosis can be overwhelming, making it difficult to absorb information and focus on what needs to be done. Your mind may be clouded with thoughts and worries about what your lung cancer will mean for you and your family. To move forward effectively, you need to make a mental adjustment. You need to redirect your energies toward the things you can control. Although you cannot change the fact that you have lung cancer, you can control how you respond to this challenge.

A first step toward gaining control of your thoughts is to realize that you are not alone in facing lung cancer. Thousands of people are surviving with lung cancer and leading happy, productive lives.

A first step toward gaining control of your thoughts is to realize that you are not alone in facing lung cancer. Thousands of people are surviving with lung cancer and leading happy, productive lives. The National Coalition for Cancer Survivorship defines a cancer survivor as anyone with a diagnosis of cancer. Cancer is not a death sentence. Many people view cancer as a chronic disease, something to be treated and managed. Keeping this concept in mind will help make your cancer experience less frightening.

Your new job is to become an involved cancer patient. The process of taking an active role in your health care will help you to gain stability, confidence, and hope. Your efforts can make a difference in the quality of your care.

Try to focus your energies on the following activities:

- *Adopting a healthy lifestyle.* Not smoking, maintaining adequate nutrition, and minimizing stress can all help your ability to fight your disease and withstand the effects of your cancer treatment (see Section 9).

- *Assembling a medical team.* You need to find doctors whom you can trust and who will provide you with excellent care. This may involve getting second opinions. You should keep in mind that good communication with all members of your medical team—including support personnel—is critical to the quality of care you receive (see Question 19).

- *Gathering information and making informed decisions.* You need to learn all you can about lung cancer and its treatment so that you will understand what is happening to you. After gathering information and discussing your treatment options with your doctor, you will be able to make informed decisions about your care.

- *Learning to navigate the healthcare system.* Your doctor's office staff and hospital social workers can help you learn how to navigate the healthcare system. This will make your appointments more productive and minimize the aggravation over medical paperwork, insurance, and financial concerns (see Questions 29 and 30).

Consider joining a patient advocacy group. There are several specific to lung cancer and you can research the various groups to find one whose mission best fits your interest (for example: research, patient support, education/awareness, legislative initiatives) (see Question 100).

26. How do I cope with the stigma of having a "self-inflicted" disease? Should I feel guilty about my smoking? What if I never smoked—how do I cope with having a "smoker's disease?"

Your emotions following your lung cancer diagnosis are likely to be complicated by your feelings about smoking. If you were an active smoker, you may experience feelings of guilt. If you never smoked, or if you had stopped smoking years before, you may be shocked that you have been diagnosed with a smoking-related disease. This personal conflict over smoking is often made worse by the reactions of those around you and by the lack of public support for people with lung cancer. Some family members and friends may be angry with you for having caused your own disease. When acquaintances learn of your lung cancer, you may get tired of hearing the inevitable question, "Did you smoke?" And it is devastating to discover that the support services, media coverage, and fundraising events that are routine for other major cancers are rare for lung cancer. This lack of public empathy and support is demoralizing and adds additional stress to the challenges you face. Thankfully, there are now several organizations such as the National Lung Cancer Partnership, working very hard to raise awareness and educate the general public about the realities of lung cancer, as well as to raise research funds.

It is important to let go of any feelings of guilt. Guilt over smoking wastes energy that could go toward fighting your disease.

It is important to let go of any feelings of guilt. Guilt over smoking wastes energy that could go toward fighting your disease. Keep in mind that smoking is legal (you have done nothing wrong) and is highly addicting. Over 90% of smokers begin smoking as teenagers, at an age when they are rebellious, feel invulnerable, and are unlikely to believe or understand the risks and addictive nature of tobacco. The tobacco companies continue to play an unconscionable role in perpetuating this deadly addiction among young people. In addition, they have specifically manufactured their cigarettes to be highly physically addictive.

It is also important to note that the majority of lung cancer diagnoses occur in a combination of former smokers (50%) and those who have never smoked (15–20%). Regardless of whether one has or hasn't smoked, no one deserves lung cancer.

One productive step you can take to help de-stigmatize this disease is to use whatever opportunities you have to put a face on lung cancer. Do not be afraid to speak up and identify yourself as a lung cancer survivor. The public needs to know that lung cancer affects everyone—mothers, fathers, sisters, brothers, and loved ones, young and old. It is easy to ignore lung cancer when "smokers" are cited as its victims. A "smoker" is an abstract notion, not a person with a life-threatening disease, worthy of caring and support. People with lung cancer are good people too—they have names, faces, and families, and they deserve the same respect afforded other cancer survivors. You can also advocate through an established organization that is dedicated to changing the perception about lung cancer (see above). For some, advocacy efforts can help the patient and/or family members focus emotional energy in a positive and hopeful way.

27. *What should I tell my children about my lung cancer? What if my children are grown?*

Lung cancer does not just affect patients; it also affects their families and friends. Children are particularly vulnerable, and their welfare is often the primary concern of parents with lung cancer. Children should be told about a parent's illness. If things are hidden from them, or they are lied to, they will at some point sense that something is wrong. This may cause them to feel isolated or to fear that things are worse than they are. There is a good chance they will discover the truth anyway—either from overhearing conversations or from an unintentional slip—causing a loss of trust between parent and child at a time when that trust is so vital. It is better if they hear the news directly from a parent, so that it can be presented in a controlled and reassuring manner. In general, learning the truth about a parent's cancer will reduce a child's fear, even if the truth is frightening. It will remove uncertainty and enable the child to learn productive ways of coping with a difficult situation.

Before discussing your lung cancer with your child, you should give what you are going to say some thought, and try to anticipate questions your child may ask.

Consider the following:

- Children need information presented in a clear, understandable manner. Appropriate information will depend on the age and emotional maturity of the child. You know your child best. In general, you do not need to tell your child every detail, but you should not lie. You can be honest about uncertainty, but try to present the information in a realistic, yet hopeful light.

- Prepare your child for what will happen next. If your child knows ahead of time that you will be having treatment and that you will experience side effects from your treatment (such as losing your hair or being very tired), he or she will be better able to adjust to your condition. It is helpful to stress that these effects are temporary.

- Reassure your child that someone will always be there to take care of him. Your child may worry about how your cancer will impact his or her life. It is important that your child's environment and activities be kept as normal as possible.

- Encourage your child to express his feelings and to ask questions. You may want to provide opportunities for your child to express his thoughts in writing or by drawing pictures.

- Let your child know that he or she may hear some frightening things about cancer, but that he should come to you to get the facts. You can tell him that while some people die from cancer, many people survive because they get effective treatments from their doctors. Stress that your doctors are taking good care of you and that you are getting the best treatments.

- Your child may want to meet your doctor. This can be a very positive experience. It can allow a child to feel more involved and to gain a more concrete understanding of what is being done to make you better. It is important that you take your cue about this from your child. No child should be forced to participate in anything beyond his or her comfort level.

- Let your child know that he or she did nothing to cause your cancer. If you smoked, you might anticipate a question about whether you caused your lung cancer by smoking.

It is a good idea to let your child's teachers (and the school psychologist, social worker and/or guidance counselor) know about your lung cancer and family situation.

It is a good idea to let your child's teachers (and the school psychologist, social worker and/or guidance counselor) know about your lung cancer and family situation. These professionals can be extremely supportive during this time and can be alert to signs that your child may need extra help to cope with his or her feelings about your cancer. You should be aware that older children need as much support as younger children, and efforts should take into account the way your child expresses herself or himself in times of distress.

If you have adult children, what you choose to share with them about your lung cancer will depend upon the nature of your relationship. You will likely find that your children will react as you would have expected, but do not be surprised if your cancer causes them to act in ways you may not have anticipated. Even as an adult, it can be overwhelming to learn that one's parent has a life-threatening illness. If you find your children acting in ways that hurt you or make you uncomfortable (such as being overprotective or becoming emotionally distant), try to express your feelings and keep the lines of communication open. This becomes especially critical when your children do not live close to you, as is often the case with grown children. In particular, you will need to work out a system for relaying important medical information. You may feel comfortable handling this yourself, or you may have the person who accompanies you to doctor visits talk to your children about medical details. In any case, you should let your doctor know which family members you would like to be involved in your care.

28. *What do caregivers need to know to best support a person with lung cancer?*

Caregivers play a vital role in the life of lung cancer patients, but they shoulder responsibilities that can be overwhelming at times. Demands placed on caregivers can be both emotionally and physically exhausting. To effectively support patients, caregivers must attend to their own needs, just as they attend to the needs of their patients. The following suggestions will help you to minimize the stress of the caregiving experience and become a more effective caregiver.

Educate yourself about lung cancer. Learn as much as you can about lung cancer, its treatments and side effects, and disease complications such as breathing distress. This will help you to understand what the patient is going through, and allow you to be a better cancer supporter and advocate.

Establish a relationship with the patient's doctor. The patient should let his doctor know that you are the primary caregiver. With the patient's permission, the doctor will answer any questions you may have. Be sure you understand your specific responsibilities for care at home (such as dispensing medication, monitoring and reporting symptoms, and managing IV and oxygen therapy), and under what circumstances you should call the doctor's office for assistance.

Seek out help for daily tasks. Don't try to go it alone. Let family and friends know the work involved in being a caregiver, and identify specific ways that they might help you, such as running errands or spending time with the patient so you can take a break. If you can delegate responsibility for managing insurance paperwork to a trusted and competent person, this will relieve you of a significant source of aggravation.

Monitor your stress and health. Be mindful of how you are feeling, and try to address issues before you become overwhelmed. Set limits for what you can do and be sure to take time away from the patient to attend to your own needs. Remember: caring for yourself is as important as caring for your loved one. If you are not healthy, the patient will suffer, too.

Keep communication open. Providing emotional support is a critical aspect of caregiving. Often it is enough just to listen. You can and should talk about your own feelings and fears about the future. If you have anger over the patient's previous or current smoking, this is not a productive time to vent. The patient needs your unconditional support. It can be useful to discuss the changes in your relationship that have come about as a result of the patient's lung cancer diagnosis.

Seek out emotional support. Find people you can talk to about your experiences. This can be good friends or other family members. It is particularly helpful to find other caregivers who share your perspective and experience. You can often find support groups for caregivers and family members at hospitals, and through organizations like CancerCare and the Wellness Community. The Association of Cancer Online Resources (ACOR) has an online support group for caregivers of people with cancer. (For further information on these resources, see the "support services" section of Question 100.) If you have persistent difficulties coping with your situation, you should seek professional counseling.

Focus on the positive. Although the challenges of caregiving are often daunting, the rewards are immeasurable. Caregiving is the greatest gift that one can give to a cancer patient. You gain the satisfaction of knowing that you actively helped your loved one in a time of need. Amidst the tedium, the aggravation, and the anguish are moments of tenderness and love that would not exist outside the cancer experience. If your loved one has limited time, you gain peace of mind that you have done the best you could to help him through his most difficult journey.

PRACTICAL ASPECTS

29. What insurance and financial concerns do I need to address following a lung cancer diagnosis?

As difficult as it is to think about, newly diagnosed cancer patients must pay immediate and careful attention to insurance and financial concerns. The costs associated with cancer care can present an enormous economic burden. For the uninsured and underinsured, this financial strain can be devastating. Even for those who are well insured, cancer-related medical expenses can cause financial hardship. Inadequate insurance and insufficient finances can have a negative impact on the amount and quality of your cancer care, and on the course of your disease. Being proactive about your financial needs can help you minimize the cost and aggravation associated with your cancer experience and will ensure that you can afford quality health care.

As difficult as it is to think about, newly diagnosed cancer patients must pay immediate and careful attention to insurance and financial concerns.

Your first step should be to examine your current health insurance coverage. Familiarize yourself with your policy and learn the scope of your medical coverage: What are your benefits? What are your restrictions? Are there circumstances under which you need pre-certification for coverage? Most physicians and/or hospitals have financial counselors who can advise you as to what the treatments will cost and what your cost or responsibility will be.

Look at the sections on how to file claims and how to appeal denied claims. Try to anticipate what your medical needs might be, including the possibility for long-term care or **hospice**. Do you have adequate coverage in your current policy? If you do not have insurance or are underinsured, there are still options available to you despite your cancer diagnosis.

Hospice

A philosophy of end-of-life care that focuses on palliative rather than curative care and provides a wide range of support to dying patients and their families.

After assessing your insurance coverage, you need to examine your financial resources. Will you be able to comfortably pay all out-of-pocket costs? There are costs associated with cancer beyond health care, such as additional transportation and childcare expenses. You must also be prepared for the possibility that you may not be able to work for an indefinite period of time. Depending on your situation, you may need to convert your life insurance policy, retirement account, or other personal property into liquid assets. Now is the time to explore all potential avenues for financial assistance. You should get sound advice, and give careful consideration, before making any financial decisions. A financial counselor is best able to advise you on your current and future financial health.

There is a wide range of resources that you can turn to for assistance with your insurance and financial needs. Some of these resources include your doctor's staff, your hospital's social worker or financial counselor, your employer's benefits manager, and nonprofit organizations such as the American Cancer Society, United Way, CancerCare, and the Patient Advocate Foundation. These individuals and organizations can help you to navigate the complex insurance and managed care systems, provide direct assistance with your paperwork or finances, or refer you to additional sources of support in your community. They can lead you to services and programs, both private and government-sponsored, that you may be eligible for and that may be useful to you.

Some of these may include:

- Additional health insurance through private carriers or government entitlement programs such as Medicare and Medicaid
- Disability benefits (private, employment, state, social security)
- Legal protections for getting and retaining health insurance coverage, preventing gaps in coverage, and for when you have been discriminated against due to your lung cancer
- Allowable medical deductions on your income taxes
- Family Medical Leave Act (FMLA)
- Veterans' Benefits
- Specialized assistance programs for patients in need who require transportation for cancer care or access to free medications

For further information on these organizations, services, and government programs, see Question 100. For an outstanding book that provides comprehensive, in-depth information on this subject, see David S. Landry's *Be Prepared: The Complete Financial, Legal, and Practical Guide to Living with Cancer, HIV, and Other Life-Challenging Conditions*, published by St. Martin's Press (1998).

COPING WITH YOUR DIAGNOSIS

30. How do I learn to manage the medical paperwork? What are medical records, and what should I know about them?

Lung cancer generates a seemingly endless stream of medical appointments and paperwork. Handling the administrative tasks associated with your cancer care takes up substantial amounts of time and adds further stress to your already difficult situation. By understanding and organizing your medical information and paperwork, you will be better equipped to manage the logistics of your cancer care. This will help save you valuable time and reduce your aggravation.

Health information generated about you by your healthcare providers and your medical facilities becomes part of your medical record. Chart notes kept by your doctor, lab tests, CT scan reports, pathology reports, consultation reports, and hospital discharge notes are all examples of medical records. Medical records are used by your providers to plan your care and to communicate with each other. They are also used by insurance companies and legal entities to document your health care. Accurate health information compiled in a timely manner is essential for quality health care. Because mistakes are not uncommon, you should obtain copies of your medical reports at the time they are generated. Copies of chart notes are usually required when applying for social security benefits. In most cases, healthcare providers and medical facilities will accommodate patient requests for copies of medical records, although they may charge a small fee. (State laws vary on patient access to medical records. You can contact your state's health department to determine your rights.) The confidentiality of your personal health information (PHI) is protected by law.

Your medical records will not be shared with third parties without your authorization.

An effective way to manage the medical information and records that you will acquire during the course of your care is to use a three-ring binder with multiple dividers. This method of organization can be tailored to your needs, and the binder can be brought with you to every medical appointment. Binder sections might include personal information, medical information (including staging and treatment details), names of healthcare providers, reports (imaging, consultation, lab), pre-testing instructions, and insurance and billing records.

In addition to paper records, you need to collect copies of your imaging films, such as x-rays and CT scans. This is best done at the time of the study. Be sure to tell the technician prior to your scan that you would like duplicate copies of the films to bring home with you. In most instances, this request is easily accommodated. In some cases, you may have a delay in getting films (from a couple of hours to a day), and you may have to pay a small fee. If they give you the actual films, they can be kept in an inexpensive portfolio, which you can purchase at any art supply store. More and more often, however, they are given to you on a computer disk or CD. Unfortunately, these tend to get lost easily. Ask if you can have a second copy made for yourself.

You may also need to get your pathology slides. These slides contain tissue specimens from your biopsy or surgery. You will need these slides when you are obtaining a second opinion. You can arrange with the hospital tissue bank or your doctor's office to obtain these yourself, or to have them sent directly to the consulting physician. It is helpful to know that the tissue bank also has your tumor block, which is an amount of your tissue left over from the operation that is generally kept for a number of years (this varies by institution), because there may be occasions when you need additional tissue specimens for further testing.

PART FIVE

What Types of Treatments Are Available for Lung Cancer?

What are the goals of treatment?

What does my surgeon mean when he or she says, "I got it all"?

What is surgery for lung cancer? How is it performed?

More . . .

31. What types of treatments are available for lung cancer?

The three traditional treatments for lung cancer include surgery, radiation therapy, and chemotherapy.

Radiotherapy

The treatment of disease with ionizing radiation. Also called radiation therapy.

Intravenous

In the vein.

Targeted therapy

Therapy directed at aspects of the cell that are specific for cancer.

The three traditional treatments for lung cancer include surgery, radiation therapy, and chemotherapy. Lung surgery commonly involves an operation to remove the tumor, along with nearby lymph nodes (see Question 34). Radiation therapy (or **radiotherapy**) is the delivery of a beam of radiation aimed at the tumor with the goal of killing some or all of the cancer cells, thus shrinking the tumor (see Question 46). Both surgery and radiotherapy are local forms of treatment, which means that they kill or remove only the tumor they are aimed at. Chemotherapy is a word for medications that kill cancer cells or stop their growth (see Question 39). Most chemotherapies are given **intravenously** (injected or dripped into the veins), but some are pills and are given orally. In either case, they get into the bloodstream and circulate around the body. Because blood flows through all parts of the body, in theory cancer cells anywhere in the body would be exposed to the chemotherapy. Therefore, chemotherapy is a systemic therapy. Recently, "**targeted therapy**" has been added as a fourth modality for lung cancer. Targeted therapies are oral or intravenous medications that "target" abnormalities found in tumors or cancer cells, but not normal tissues. Although targeted therapies are "systemic" treatments, like chemotherapy, they tend to have fewer side effects because they do not affect normal cells. Some examples of targeted therapies include bevacizumab (Avastin) or erlotinib (Tarceva).

New treatments for lung cancer are always being tested in research studies known as clinical trials. You should familiarize yourself with the advantages and disadvantages of participation in clinical trials and explore the treatment options available to you through clinical trials (see Questions 59 and 60). If you are considering alternative therapies, such as herbal therapies, you should have an understanding of how to evaluate them. Alternative therapies are treatments not endorsed by the traditional medical establishment because their effectiveness and safety have not been proven in rigorous scientific studies (see Question 61).

32. What are the goals of treatment?

For patients with early stage (Stage I–IIIA) cancer, the goals of treatment are usually cure. **Curative treatment** is just what it sounds like—treatment given in order to cure the patient of his or her cancer. Typically, curative treatment for non-small cell lung cancer will include surgery, if the disease was discovered at an early stage. For Stage III disease (see Question 56), curative treatment may consist of chemotherapy and surgery, or chemotherapy and radiation therapy. For a limited stage small cell lung cancer, curative treatment usually consists of a combination of both chemotherapy and radiation therapy to the tumor in the chest.

Realistically, treatment of advanced, metastatic lung cancer is usually not curative. Instead, the goals of treatment are to prolong survival, shrink the tumor if at all possible, and improve the symptoms from the tumor. Chemotherapy is administered with the intent to shrink the tumor or at least keep it stable and stop it from growing. In doing so, one hopes to prolong life and decrease symptoms, thereby improving quality of life.

Palliation usually refers to treatments which are directed at reducing symptoms. Radiation therapy is an example of a treatment that can be either curative or palliative. Sometimes, high doses of radiation therapy can be

Curative treatment

Treatment given with the intent to cure the patient of his or her cancer.

Palliation

Reducing symptoms.

administered with curative intent to lung cancer patients with local disease who are not candidates for surgery. More commonly, however, somewhat lower doses of radiation therapy ("palliative" doses) are administered to shrink a tumor that is causing symptoms, such as metastases that have spread to the brain, spinal cord, and bone. Occasionally, it is also given to the primary tumor in the chest. Palliative radiation is usually effective at reducing the neurological signs and symptoms from the brain metastasis; reducing pain from the bone metastasis and preventing bone fractures; and improving tumor-related symptoms, such as shortness of breath, cough, or bleeding.

It is appropriate to ask your doctor about the goals of treatment if he or she has not already told you.

Performance status

The general condition of the patient.

The general sense of well-being of the patient is an important prognostic factor; that is, patients who have relatively few symptoms are more likely to do well than patients who are very fatigued, weak, anorexic, and losing weight.

33. What is performance status, and why is it important?

Performance status is a term used to describe the general condition of the patient. The general sense of well-being of the patient is an important prognostic factor; that is, patients who have relatively few symptoms are more likely to do well than patients who are very fatigued, weak, anorexic, and losing weight. Several different grading systems for performance status are currently used, including the ECOG (Eastern Cooperative Oncology Group) grading system and the Zubrich grading system. The ECOG grading system is rated on a scale of 0 to 4 and is defined in **Table 2**. The Zubrich grading system is defined on a scale of 100% to 0%, where 100% is totally asymptomatic and 0% is very near death.

Performance status is often used in defining eligibility for a clinical trial (see Question 59). Because patients

Table 2 ECOG PS Grading System

PS	GRADE DESCRIPTION
0	Totally asymptomatic
1	Mildly symptomatic, able to perform daily activities
2	Able to perform daily activities with assistance, spends less than 50% of the day in bed
3	Needs considerable assistance for performing daily activities, spends greater than 50% of the day in bed
4	Totally bed-ridden, unable to care for oneself

with poor performance status are often very weak, most clinical trials exclude patients with a performance status of 2 through 4. There is, however, increasing interest in defining treatment for these patients as well.

SURGERY

34. What is surgery for lung cancer? How is it performed?

Ideally, surgery for lung cancer should be done by a thoracic surgeon (see Question 18). The type of surgery performed depends upon the stage of tumor, and the medical condition of the patient. The most typical operation is a lobectomy and mediastinal **lymph node dissection**. A **lobectomy** is the removal of the lobe of the lung in which the tumor is located. A mediastinal lymph node dissection consists of removing some or all of the mediastinal lymph nodes (the lymph nodes between the lung and heart). This is often done to determine whether the tumor has spread to these lymph nodes. Occasionally, a patient may be unable to tolerate a lobectomy

Lymph node dissection

Surgical removal of lymph nodes.

Lobectomy

Surgical removal of a lobe of the lung.

because underlying bronchitis or emphysema ("COPD") makes it too difficult for the remaining lung to keep the person alive. In these cases, a surgeon will sometimes do a **wedge resection**. This consists of removing the tumor and a small amount of lung tissue surrounding the tumor, but not the whole lobe. A wedge resection will preserve more normal lung, but the chances of the cancer coming back are somewhat higher.

Wedge resection

Surgical removal of the tumor and a small amount of lung tissue surrounding the tumor.

Occasionally, the tumor is located in an area such that all the lobes of the lung on that side are involved, meaning that they all contain some tumor. Sometimes the tumor is located in the largest airway on that side (the right or left main stem bronchus, which is the first major division of the trachea, the air pipe that delivers air to the lungs). If one of the main stem bronchi is involved, or if the tumor involves all the lobes on one side, a **pneumonectomy** must be performed. In a pneumonectomy, the whole lung is removed. Obviously, this is a much bigger procedure than a lobectomy or a wedge resection. Although a person with two normal lungs should be able to tolerate removal of one of the lungs without a major impact on his or her breathing, very often patients who have been smoking and have a substantial amount of emphysema or bronchitis are not able to tolerate a pneumonectomy.

Pneumonectomy

Surgical removal of the entire lung.

Typically, lung surgery involves an operation called a **thoracotomy**, which requires the surgeon to make a large incision in the chest to gain access to the lungs. Less invasive surgical techniques, such as video-assisted thoracoscopic surgery ("VATS"), involve smaller incisions and hold promise for reduced post-operative pain and complications and shorter hospital stays.

Thoracotomy

A common type of lung surgery that requires a large incision to provide access to the lungs.

35. What determines whether I am able to have surgery?

To determine whether a patient is a candidate for surgery, three things must be established first:

1. Has the cancer metastasized? If the cancer has spread to other organs (Stage IV), a surgical cure is not possible and it does not make sense to do a large operation, considering the side effects, cost, and risks associated with surgery. Therefore, patients with metastatic disease usually do not undergo a curative resection.

2. The tumor must be **resectable**—that is, located in a place that the surgeon will be able to get to and completely remove. For example, if the tumor involves the heart, the surgeon obviously cannot safely remove the heart, and the tumor would be considered unresectable. In general, a tumor is considered unresectable if it involves any other major structures in the center of the chest, such as the heart, the large blood vessels going in and out of the heart, or the windpipe leading from the mouth to the lungs (the trachea).

3. The third criterion for surgery is that a patient must be healthy enough to withstand it. In particular, this involves two organs—the heart and the lungs:

   a. *The heart.* If you have a history of heart disease, such as congestive heart failure, angina, or heart attacks, your surgeon will want to make sure that it is safe to operate on you, so that the stress of the surgery will not result in a heart attack. He or she may ask you to see a cardiologist, or heart doctor. The cardiologist will take

Resectable

Able to be surgically removed (resected).

WHAT TYPES OF TREATMENTS ARE AVAILABLE FOR LUNG CANCER?

a history, examine you, and may order an EKG, echocardiogram, or stress test before giving a final recommendation.

b. *The lungs.* Many patients with lung cancer are smokers or former smokers, and have some degree of emphysema or bronchitis (also known as chronic obstructive pulmonary disease, or COPD). If your doctor suspects you may have COPD, he or she will order **pulmonary function tests** (PFTs). PFTs are a series of breathing tests that can help determine how healthy your lungs are and whether your remaining lungs will be able to support you if a portion of one of them has been removed. Your doctor may also order a preoperative quantitative perfusion scan, which is a nuclear medicine scan designed to predict how much lung function you will be left with after the operation.

36. What can I expect before surgery and what can I do to prepare for it?

If you are a current smoker, the most important thing you can do to prepare for surgery is stop smoking. Regardless of whether you decide to quit permanently, stopping even if only for a few days or weeks in advance will markedly improve your ability to tolerate the operation. This cannot be stressed enough. Many thoracic surgeons will not operate on a patient who is still actively smoking because of the higher risks associated with the surgery.

Prior to the operation, your surgeon will explain the procedure to you and arrange for an interview with either the anesthesiologist or a nurse anesthetist, who will go over your past medical history. You should be sure to disclose all of your medications at this time (including

Pulmonary function tests (PFTs)

A group of breathing tests used to determine lung health.

If you are a current smoker, the most important thing you can do to prepare for surgery is stop smoking.

supplements, herbs, and over-the-counter drugs) so that the anesthesiologist can determine whether you need to stop taking them before surgery. Depending upon your health, the extent of the operation, and your hospital's policy, you may be admitted the night before the procedure. Many patients, however, come to the hospital the morning of the operation. You will be brought to the pre-op surgical suite, where you will change into a gown, and an intravenous catheter (an "IV") will be inserted into your arm. You may be given a medication to help you relax. (Keep in mind that this is something you can ask for if you are feeling overly anxious.) You will then be placed on a moveable cot (or gurney) and wheeled into the operating room. At first glance, this might appear to be a cold, sterile place where everyone is wearing surgical gowns, masks, and hats. The surgical staff, however, will try to see that you are comfortable, and you will be able to talk to them. Once you are on the surgical table, the anesthesiologist will give you some medication into your vein to make you go to sleep. A tube will then be placed into your throat into which oxygen will be blown while you are asleep. You will sleep during the entire operation and wake up in the recovery room.

37. What does my surgeon mean when he or she says they "got it all"? Does this mean I am cured?

When your surgeon says she "got it all," what she is really saying is that she removed all the cancer she could see. Unfortunately, that does not necessarily mean a cure. We know that in many patients the cancer will come back—either at the original site, or elsewhere in the body. Presumably, some cancer cells that were too small for the surgeon to see or for any scans to pick up must have escaped before the operation.

Positive margins

A phrase used when cancer cells are found at the edge of the biopsy sample.

Negative margins

A phrase used when normal tissue is found at the edge of the biopsy sample.

The pathologist will look to see whether the biopsy tumor from your surgery has "**positive margins**." Positive margins mean that the cancer cells extend to the very edge of the biopsy or surgical sample. If so, there is a high likelihood that there were tumor cells remaining on the other side of the sample—i.e., the side remaining in the patient. Even if your resected tumor has "**negative margins**" (normal tissue at the edge of the biopsy sample), there is no way to determine if there were microscopic amounts of cancer cells left behind either in the area of the tumor or somewhere else in the body. Unfortunately, none of the blood tests, x-rays, or scans currently available are able to detect microscopic amounts of disease.

Many patients whose cancer recurs after surgery are confused and angry because they remember their surgeons saying they "got it all." It is important to be aware that if your surgeon says she "got it all," she does not mean "there are no longer any cancer cells in your body, and you are cured." Although there is a considerable amount of research going on to detect smaller and smaller amounts of tumor, at this point the most accurate answer to the question "did the surgeon get it all?" is "we do not know."

Keep in mind that although successful lung surgery is reason to celebrate, you need to be vigilant about your follow-up care (see Question 91).

38. What should I expect following my surgery? What are the common complications of lung surgery?

When you wake up in the recovery room, you will be very "woozy" and might not realize where you are, or even that the operation is over. You will doze off and on while you are brought back to your room. If possible, it is often helpful to have a family member or loved one stay with you during those first few days. He or she can call the nurses for you, help make you comfortable, and assist you in getting around.

For the first 24 to 48 hours, you may be uncomfortable, but the nurses should respond to your request for pain medications. Ask your doctor if you can have **patient-controlled analgesia (PCA)**, a method by which you can regulate your own pain medication. By pressing a button attached to an IV, you can give yourself a small dose of morphine whenever you need it, so that you do not have to wait for a nurse. The PCA machine is set so that you will not be able to overdose yourself.

Patient-controlled analgesia (PCA)

A method by which a patient can regulate the amount of pain medication he or she receives.

You most likely will have a chest tube when you come out of surgery. This is a tube leading from the space between your lung and chest wall to a bag or container by your bedside. Suction is applied to drain the fluid and inflate the lung. Fortunately, this is not as painful or uncomfortable as it sounds! In addition, you will probably have a catheter leading from your bladder to a bag by the bedside (a "Foley catheter"). This is also painless and will drain your bladder until you are able to go to the bathroom by yourself. Most likely, you will also have oxygen prongs or a face mask for oxygen.

Despite the IVs and catheters, the nurse will get you up out of bed the first day following your surgery. This is very important to prevent post-op complications, such as blood clots and lung problems. A lung that is not breathing normally is very susceptible to accumulation of secretions, which in turn leads to accumulation of bacteria and pneumonia. In addition, the nurse or respiratory therapist will give you lung exercises to do to prevent this

Despite the IVs and catheters, the nurse will get you up out of bed the first day following your surgery. This is very important to prevent post-op complications, such as blood clots and lung problems.

complication. It is important to have adequate pain control so that you feel like doing these exercises, so be sure to ask for and use pain medications as necessary.

You will not be allowed to eat or drink until the doctors are sure your stomach and intestines have "woken up" following the surgery. Typically, a patient's GI tract tends to stop working for several days following a general anesthesia. When you start passing gas from below, you will be allowed to drink clear liquids. Your diet will advance as your stomach and small intestine become more active.

The most common complication following lung surgery is infection—usually a lung infection, often from not breathing deeply and/or clearing secretions out of the lungs. Other unlikely complications are bleeding, infections of the incision site, and post-operative heart problems, such as congestive heart failure or an irregular heart rhythm.

Make sure that you have adequate pain medications to take home. It is not uncommon for surgeons to underestimate post-op pain. Patients are often sent home with a small supply of pain medication when, in reality, many will need to take some medications for a month or longer. If your doctor does not want to give you a large supply, make sure you know how to contact him or her for refills.

CHEMOTHERAPY

39. What is chemotherapy? How does it work?

Chemotherapy is a word for medications used to treat cancer. Unlike surgery and radiation, which are used to treat localized disease (i.e., in the lungs), chemotherapy is a systemic therapy used to treat disease that has spread to all parts of the body. Chemotherapy drugs are often administered intravenously (sometimes orally), and thus are absorbed into the blood. Since the blood flows to all parts of the body, in theory, cancer cells anywhere in the body would be exposed to the chemotherapy.

Chemotherapy works by interfering with the DNA of cancer cells (see Question 2). Because cancer cells divide rapidly and don't stop ("uncontrolled growth"), many chemotherapy drugs are specifically designed to target rapidly dividing cells. However, some normal cells in the body also grow rapidly—such as hair, the lining of the stomach, and blood cells—and chemotherapy affects these cells as well, causing unpleasant effects such as hair loss, nausea (rarely vomiting), and susceptibility to infections. Ask your doctor about ways to prevent or reduce these side effects.

Chemotherapy sometimes consists of one drug, but more often it involves a combination of drugs called a **regimen**. Chemotherapy regimens combine drugs that have different mechanisms of action, or ways of attacking cancer cells, in order to increase their effectiveness and to prevent the cancer cells from developing resistance to chemotherapy. Your doctor will recommend possible chemotherapy regimens based on your type of lung cancer, your stage, the location of your disease, your

Regimen

Specific chemotherapy treatment plan; involving the drugs, doses, and frequency of administration.

general health, any previous treatments, the side effects of the drugs, and the goals of your treatment plan. For information on specific chemotherapy drugs and regimens used to treat lung cancer, (see **Table 3**).

Above all, please note that the chemotherapy that is used to treat one type of cancer, such as breast cancer, colon cancer or prostate cancer, is very different from the chemotherapy used to treat lung cancer, and the side effects will be much different. Although support groups are very helpful in supporting you during your treatment, the side effects that some of the patients with other cancers have experienced are likely to be very different than the side effects experienced by lung cancer patients. In addition, there are many different chemotherapy regimens for lung cancers. These have different side effects, too. For example, some are more likely to cause hair loss than others. PLEASE talk to your doctor and/or nurse to get a realistic view of what YOU are likely to experience.

40. What can I expect during chemotherapy?

Complete blood count (CBC)

A blood test that counts the number of white blood cells, red blood cells, and platelets.

Phlebotomist

A technician trained to draw blood.

The typical chemotherapy session begins with a standard blood test called a **complete blood count (CBC)**. Because chemotherapy may lower your blood counts, your oncologist wants to be sure that your blood counts are high enough so that you are able to receive chemotherapy safely. (see Question 71 for a full explanation of how chemotherapy affects your blood.) You can ask your nurse or **phlebotomist** (a technician trained to draw blood) to use a small needle for your blood draw, which will minimize the discomfort caused when the needle is inserted into your vein.

The process of delivering IV chemotherapy is called an infusion. The most common IV method uses a thin needle or catheter (tiny plastic tube) that is inserted into a vein in your arm or hand. These IV needle sticks cause a bit more discomfort than a needle stick for a blood test because they require a slightly larger needle—the pain is a little sharper, but just as fleeting. Some patients apply a numbing cream (Emla) prior to needle sticks to make the process virtually painless. You may want to ask your oncologist or oncology nurse if this might be an option for you.

Once inserted, the needle or catheter is taped down to prevent it from moving and causing any pain. The chemotherapy drug(s)—and any pre-medications—are then dispensed from bags suspended from a metal IV pole. These liquids flow from the bags through a flexible tube that feeds into the needle or catheter in your vein. An infusion pump is sometimes used to deliver a precise amount of medication over a set period of time.

You will receive your pre-medications (pre-meds) first. These will likely include fluids for hydration and anti-emetics to prevent nausea and vomiting. Your oncology nurse should clearly explain the pre-meds and chemotherapy drugs you are getting. When the drugs begin to flow, you may feel a slight coldness or strange sensation at the IV site; however, the infusion process should be pain-free and uneventful. If you experience pain, burning, swelling, shortness of breath, or any other unusual reactions during your infusion, you should bring it to your nurse's attention immediately. Your nurse will check to see if the needle was inserted properly, or perhaps adjust the flow of the medication to a more comfortable rate. There are other measures that can be taken to alleviate discomfort or other problems you may experience, so you need to keep your nurse informed of your status.

The process of delivering IV chemotherapy is called an infusion. The most common IV method uses a thin needle or catheter (tiny plastic tube) that is inserted into a vein in your arm or hand.

The length of your infusion will depend on the number and amount of chemotherapy drugs you are receiving. Chemo sessions can take one hour, several hours, or several days. Extended infusions may require a hospital stay. For the duration of your infusion, it often helps to watch TV, read a book, listen to music, talk to a friend, sleep—do whatever relaxes you and makes the time go more quickly. You are unlikely to experience any side effects during the infusion. When your infusion is over, be sure your nurse has told you about any potential side effects, what to do if you experience them, and under what circumstances you should call your doctor's office. If your nurse tells you that you may experience nausea, don't leave the office without a prescription for medications to prevent nausea and be sure you know how to use them.

In some instances, chemotherapy can be administered outside an office or hospital setting. For example, oral chemotherapies—in pill, capsule, or liquid form—can be taken by patients at home. Portable infusion pumps allow some IV chemotherapies to be delivered at home as patients go about their usual activities

41. What is a CVC or central line? What is a port? How do I know if I need one?

Patients typically receive chemotherapy intravenously through a thin needle that is inserted into a vein in the arm or hand. There are devices available called central venous catheters (CVCs) that are semi-permanent IVs. They may remain in for extended periods of time (often months) and allow repeated access to larger veins without the pain or stress associated with IV needle sticks into the smaller, more delicate veins. CVCs require minor surgery for insertion, but can be left in place indefinitely. There are two basic types of CVCs: external CVCs and ports (subcutaneous CVCs).

External CVCs. You may hear other patients talk about Broviac, Groshong, or Hickman catheters. These are names of common external CVCs. External CVCs are IVs which are inserted in a large blood vessel, but the other end is exposed through the skin and "capped off" so that one does not have to carry an IV bag around all the time. This allows for a convenient and pain-free IV for drawing blood and for delivering chemotherapy. They can also be used for blood transfusions, CT contrast, fluids, and nutrition. External CVCs require some care so that they won't become blocked by a blood clot or become infected. The risk of developing a blood clot can be reduced with the use of coumadin, a blood thinning medication.

Ports. Another option for convenient venous access is a port—also known as a medi-port or port-a-cath (**Figure 2**). A port is a type of **central venous catheter** that is implanted wholly under the skin. Ports provide access

External CVCs

IVs inserted in a large blood vessel. The other end is exposed through the skin and "capped off" so a patient does not have to carry an IV bag with them all the time.

Port

A type of central venous catheter that is surgically implanted under the skin.

Central venous catheter (CVC)

A thin tube that is surgically inserted to allow access to large veins.

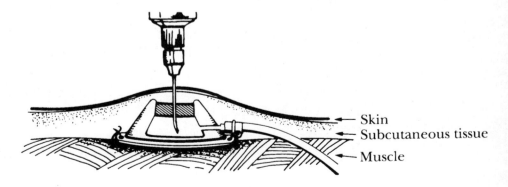

Figure 2   Schematic drawing of an implantable port.

Reprinted from Yarbro CH, Frogge MH, Goodman M, Groenwald SL: *Cancer Nursing: Principles and Practice*, Sixth Ed. Copyright © 2005, Jones and Bartlett Publishers, LLC.

to major veins but are not exposed through the skin as are external devices. They require much less care and carry less risk of infection than external CVCs. Although needle sticks must still be made through the skin, the discomfort is less than with an IV needle stick because a special needle is used, and the skin over the port toughens and becomes less sensitive over time. Numbing cream (Emla) can be applied to make this process completely pain-free. Unlike external CVCs, ports are minimally noticeable—they appear only as a small raised area under the skin. Ports require general anesthesia for insertion.

Neither external CVCs nor ports should significantly impact or change your daily activities.

Neither external CVCs nor ports should significantly impact or change your daily activities. You can still bathe and exercise, for example, and neither is noticeable under clothing. Patients who should consider getting a venous access device include:

- Patients who experience difficulty with blood drawing or chemotherapy IVs;
- Patients who will be receiving chemotherapy on a frequent basis; and
- Patients who will be receiving chemotherapy drugs irritating to small veins.

If you think you might benefit from having a venous access device such as an external CVC or a port, you should discuss this possibility with your oncologist. Most patients find that these devices greatly increase their quality of life during chemotherapy.

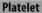

42. Why does my doctor order blood tests during my chemotherapy treatment? (see also Question 71)

Because chemotherapy attacks rapidly growing cells, it can affect your blood cells, which are among the most rapidly dividing cells in your body. This is one of the most common side effects of chemotherapy. Your blood contains white blood cells, red blood cells, and **platelets**, each of which has a specific function. If your chemotherapy treatment causes your blood counts (the number of your blood cells) to drop below normal, this can put you at risk for potentially dangerous side effects. In some cases, these effects can be prevented or controlled through the use of supportive therapies. Please note that some drugs cause more **myelosuppression** (drop in the blood counts) than others (see Table 3). Also, some drugs may affect one type of blood cell more than others. For example, while almost all drugs affect the white blood cells, Gemzar (gemcitabine) and carboplatin also lower the platelet count.

Platelet

A type of blood cell responsible for clotting.

Myelo-suppression

A decrease in the production of blood cells.

The drop in blood counts is usually temporary. The counts are often at their lowest between 10 to 14 days after the chemotherapy, at which point they start to bounce back. The counts are usually back to normal by the time the next treatment is to be delivered.

43. What are the common side effects of chemotherapy? (see also Part 7)

Although all chemotherapy has side effects, the reality is that most lung cancer patients tolerate chemotherapy relatively well. In fact, tales of nausea and vomiting—among the most feared effects of chemotherapy—date from years ago when chemotherapy drugs were more toxic and when

Antiemetics

Drugs that prevent nausea and vomiting.

Alopecia

Hair loss.

Peripheral neuropathy

Tingling, numbness, or burning sensation in hands, feet, or legs caused by damage to peripheral nerves by a tumor or by chemotherapy or radiation.

effective anti-nausea drugs (**antiemetics**) were not available. Advances in medicine have led to the development of chemotherapy drugs with fewer and less severe side effects. Oncologists can now provide patients with supportive therapies such as antiemetic drugs to prevent nausea and vomiting, medications to control pain, and growth factors to restore blood counts. It is important to remember that there is always something that can be done to eliminate, reduce, or help you cope with side effects from chemotherapy. The one possible exception is hair loss (**alopecia**). There are no effective ways to decrease hair loss by drugs that cause it, although not all chemotherapy drugs cause hair loss.

A comforting thought is that almost all chemotherapy side effects are temporary and resolve immediately following treatment. It helps to remind yourself of this whenever you are experiencing distressing effects. Infrequently, there can be side effects that persist after treatment and never go away completely. Patients who experience severe **peripheral neuropathy**, for example, often complain that they have residual tingling and numbness in their fingers and toes years after chemotherapy. There are also a small number of side effects that may appear after treatment is completed—so-called "late effects." Although rare, these can be serious (for example, second cancers are considered "late effects") and should be discussed with your oncologist prior to treatment. (See Question 79 for additional information on long-term and late effects.)

For additional information on side effects, see Part 7, Side Effects of Chemotherapy.

44. What is "targeted therapy"?

Unlike chemotherapy, which kills both normal (e.g., hair cells or blood cells) and cancer cells indiscriminately, many of these newer treatments are targeted at aspects of the cell that are specific for cancer—hence the term targeted therapies. Many of these drugs try to stop or inhibit chemical reactions, sometimes called pathways, which are active only in cancer cells and not normal cells. Interestingly, for many of these chemical reactions to occur, the pathway must *be activated* by a signal (or **ligand**) coming from outside the cell. This signal, or ligand, does not diffuse into the cell. Instead, it binds to a molecule on the surface of the cell called a **receptor**. When this happens, the receptor becomes activated, and starts the cascade of chemical reactions which eventually gets to the nucleus and activated abnormal, mutated genes. A theoretical advantage of these targeted therapies is that because they are specific for cancer cells and should not affect normal ones, the side effects associated with them should be much less. Indeed this is the case; these drugs rarely cause hair loss, nausea, or a drop in the blood counts.

Two major classes of drugs make up targeted therapies—antibodies and small molecules. The antibodies used for cancer are similar to the antibodies our bodies make to help fight infection. However, instead of attacking bacteria, these man-made antibodies attack very specific molecules called receptors on the outside surface of the cancer cell, and in doing so, block certain functions. Antibodies are almost always given IV. Because our bodies will recognize them as "foreign," they are sometimes associated with allergic ("hypersensitivity") reactions.

Ligand

An ion, a molecule, or a molecular group that binds to another chemical entity to form a larger complex.

Receptor

A protein molecule, embedded in either the plasma membrane or cytoplasm of a cell, to which a mobile signaling (or "signal") molecule may attach.

Small molecules, on the other hand, are just what they sound like—molecules which are much smaller than antibodies, and are made to block specific "pathways," or chemical reactions, on the inside of the cancer cell. Many of them are given in pill form. One type of small molecule you may hear about is called "tyrosine kinase inhibitors" or "TKIs." TKIs block the activated part of the receptor on the inside of the cell, and prevent it from starting the chain reaction.

In many cases, there are antibodies and small molecules which target the same pathway. In some instances, it is not known which is better—the antibody or the small molecule.

A number of different areas of investigation can be lumped under the term "targeted therapies." Two general categories which are approved for the treatment for lung cancer include:

Growth factor inhibitors

Substances that inhibit the growth factors that stimulate cells to grow.

- **Growth factor inhibitors.** As mentioned in Question 2, cancer cells are often stimulated to grow by substances called growth factors. One of particular interest is the epidermal growth factor (EGF). EGF is probably made by some cancer cells, and is secreted into the space surrounding the cancer cell and the rest of the cancer cells that make up the tumor. In doing this, the EGF-secreting cancer cell stimulates its neighbors to grow. The EGF doesn't directly diffuse into a cell; instead, it binds to a receptor on the outside of the cell. Binding of the EGF to the EGF receptor (EGFR) activates the receptor, causing a chemical chain reaction that eventually ends up in the nucleus of the cell, stimulating the cell to grow.

A number of different drugs are being developed to stop EGF from activating the receptor, and/or stopping the chain reaction that tells the DNA to start to grow and divide. Some of these drugs work by blocking the EGF from getting to the receptor (these are usually antibodies to the receptor and come in IV form; cetuximab or Erbitux is an example); others work by preventing the activated receptor from sending chemical signals to the nucleus. Tarceva (erlotinib) is an example of this latter kind of drug, which usually comes in oral form. At this point, it is not known whether either approach is better than the other. However, Tarceva is rarely given at the same time as chemotherapy ("concurrently"), whereas Erbitux is rarely given alone.

It is not clear which patients may benefit from one of the EGFR inhibitors. Obviously, if your tumor doesn't have EGFR, you do not have the "target" for these "targeted drugs," and it would seem unlikely you would benefit. However, nearly everyone (85%–90%) has EGFR, and yet not everyone benefits, so scientists are studying the tumors to see if they can predict who is likely to respond. Patients who have a mutation in their EGFR are very likely to have a response, but only about 10% of North Americans and Europeans are likely to have a mutation. Patients whose tumors have a lot of receptor ("over-expression") may benefit as well.

- **Angiogenesis inhibitors.** As discussed in Question 2, tumors need a constant and growing blood supply to feed them, much like an advancing army needs a constant and growing supply of food and materials to sustain it. Blocking off this blood supply should, in theory, have two effects: it should "choke off" the cancer by stopping the flow of oxygen and nutrients to it, and it should stop the tumor from

Angiogenesis inhibitors

Drugs that prevent the formation of new blood vessels.

spreading through its usual highway—the bloodstream. Avastin, or bevacizumab, is the first of these agents approved for lung cancer. Avastin is an antibody, similar to the antibodies that block the EGF pathway mentioned above. However, Avastin blocks a growth signal called **VEGF (vascular endothelial growth factor)** from binding to its receptor on the surface of blood vessel cells, not cancer cells. VEGF stimulates the blood vessel cells (endothelial cells) to grow, divide, and migrate into the tumor. As with the EGF pathway, a number of small molecules or TKIs are being developed which work by preventing the activated receptor from sending chemical signals to the nucleus. This is a promising area of cancer research, with many new and ongoing clinical trials in lung cancer.

VEGF (vascular endothelial growth factor)

A sub-family of growth factors, more specifically of platelet-derived growth factor family of cystine-knot growth factors.

45. What are common side effects of targeted therapies?

Major side effects of EGFR inhibitors such as Tarceva (erlotinib) or Erbitux (cetuximab) are rash, and less commonly, diarrhea. The rash looks like acne, and is typically scattered over the trunk and face. In some patients, it can be severe. If you develop a severe rash, talk to your doctor. He or she will probably prescribe antibiotics and may reduce your dose.

A common side effect of angiogenesis inhibitors is hypertension. Your doctor should be monitoring you for high blood pressure and, if need be, giving you blood pressure medications, or adding to or changing the ones you are currently on. Another somewhat less common side effect is the loss of very small amounts of protein in the urine. Your physician may ask you to give periodic urine samples to check for this. A rare side effect of these drugs is coughing up blood, particularly in patients with squamous cell carcinoma. If this happens to you, notify your doctor at once because, very rarely, some patients with squamous cell carcinoma have died of this complication. Because of this, Avastin is limited to patients without squamous cell carcinoma, and those with no history of coughing up blood. Some doctors will also withhold Avastin or other angiogenic inhibitors from patients with large tumors that are located next to large blood vessels, although this has not been definitely shown to be a risk factor for bleeding.

RADIATION THERAPY

46. What is radiation therapy?

Radiation therapy (also sometimes referred to as radiotherapy, x-ray therapy, irradiation, or cobalt) is the use of high-energy rays to stop cancer cells from growing or multiplying.

47. How does radiation work?

Radiation affects normal and abnormal cells in the area being treated. It causes damage to the DNA, which is often permanent, causing cells to die. After cell death, the cellular remains must eventually disintegrate and be removed from the body. This dead cell removal may be quite slow and there may be a delay in the shrinkage of tumors receiving radiation, even though all the cells are dead.

Radiation treatment is carefully planned to deliver as much radiation as possible to tumor cells while doing as little damage as possible to normal surrounding cells.

Radiation treatment is carefully planned to deliver as much radiation as possible to tumor cells while doing as little damage as possible to normal surrounding cells.

Radiation is usually given in small doses over a long period of time to increase the effect on the tumor cells while providing intervals between treatments to allow injured normal tissues to recover, thus reducing the side effects of radiation.

48. What is a "dose" of radiation? How many treatments will I need?

The "dose" of radiation is measured in units called **rads** or **Gray (Gy)**. The typical dose of radiation is about 6000 rads or 60 Gy. (This is also equivalent to 6000 **centigray**, because one Gy = 100 centigray.) Rather than administer all 60 Gy in one treatment, the radiation is divided up into many treatments. The total dose of radiation and the number of treatments you will need will depend on the size, location, and type of your cancer.

Radiation delivered with "curative" intent usually consists of about 60 Gy given 2 Gy at a time, in 30 treatments or **fractions**. Treatments are typically given daily, although occasionally specific reasons require that treatment be given more frequently (twice a day) or less frequently (two to three times a week). Usually, radiation is given five days a week, Monday through Friday, over six weeks. Some data suggest that, in certain situations, giving the radiation therapy twice per day for a total of 12 days may be more effective than the standard schedule.

Radiation oncologists are also developing ways to give even higher doses of radiation (70 Gy or higher) without damaging surrounding tissue. When delivered to the brain, for example, it is sometimes given by a device called the "gamma knife" or the "cyber knife" (depending upon the type of device) or radiosurgery.

Rad

Unit of radiation.

Gray (Gy)

Modern unit of radiation dosage (100 rads is equal to one Gy).

Centigray

Unit of radiation; same as a rad.

Fraction

Single treatment of radiation. The total dose of radiation is usually given over multiple fractions.

The amount of radiation given to reduce symptoms ("palliative" radiation) is usually less than what is given in an attempt to cure the patient. This is because smaller doses of radiation can shrink the tumor enough to reduce symptoms and have fewer side effects than "high dose" radiation.

49. What equipment is used to deliver radiation?

A variety of specialized equipment is used in both planning and treatment with radiation therapy. An x-ray machine called a simulator is used during the planning phase. A computer may also be used. The simulator and computer help determine the best plan for the area which needs to be treated (**"treatment fields"**).

Treatment field

The area of the body which is radiated.

The treatment may be delivered with linear accelerators or cobalt accelerators. Modern advances in the linear accelerator have made it the most commonly used equipment. A linear accelerator or **"linac"** produces high-energy x-rays. Instead of x-rays, the cobalt machines produce a different type of energy beam called gamma rays. X-rays and gamma rays are very similar. One machine is chosen over the other based on technical factors of the machines and not on any difference in the effectiveness of the radiation beams in destroying cancer cells. The radiation oncologist's decision about which radiation-producing equipment to use is based on many factors, such as the type of cancer and its particular location in the patient.

Linac

A linear accelerator which produces high energy x-rays for radiation therapy.

50. What can I expect during radiation therapy?

Your first visit to the radiation therapy department lasts one to three hours and usually does not include any treatments. A radiation oncologist will review your records and examine you to decide whether radiation therapy is appropriate and which treatment plan is best. He or she will discuss treatment recommendations with you, including how many treatments are needed and what their effects are likely to be. This is the time to ask questions. Your next appointment will be for a treatment planning CT or a **simulation** and you may not see the doctor.

Simulation

Planning the radiation fields with a CT scan.

The purpose of the simulation visit is to plan the technical aspects of your treatments. A therapist will take you to the simulator room where he or she will accurately plan your radiation treatments. Simulators are not treatment machines; they are specialized machines built to mimic x-ray treatment units, and to take moving or still x-ray pictures. During your simulation, x-rays may be taken. In some cases a computerized tomography (CT) simulator is used to further refine treatment planning.

A variety of methods is used to line up your treatment field correctly. A special mold may be made for you to lie in during your treatment. Tiny dots may be tattooed on your skin to mark the center and corners of your field. These look like tiny freckles and will not be visible to anyone except those who know where to look. Oil-based markers or ink may also be used to mark your skin. It is important that you do not wash the marks off until all the treatments are completed. These marks stay on best if they are not allowed to get wet for the first 24 hours; after that, you can bathe or shower. The water can run over the marks, but you should not use soap or a washcloth on the marked area. When the marks fade, the therapist touches them up at the treatment unit. The markings will rub off on clothes, so it's recommended that you wear older clothing. Pretreating the garment with a stain remover or hair spray before washing will generally remove the stain.

This simulation planning session usually takes one to two hours. You might get a treatment on this day, depending on whether special blocks need to be made for your treatment and whether there is an opening in the treatment schedule.

Most patients are treated on an outpatient basis. If you live too far away from the radiation center to commute from home, you might consider staying with local friends or relatives, or in a nearby motel. Many hospitals have arrangements with nearby motels for a lower cost for their radiation patients. The treatment schedule can generally be tailored to accommodate at least a part-time work schedule.

51. What is the actual procedure like?

Radiotherapy treatments are very similar to having x-rays. Just as you are not able to see, feel, or hear the rays in a chest x-ray, there is no pain or discomfort with the actual radiation treatment. If you are in pain for other reasons, the treatment process may be uncomfortable because you will be required to lie still for a short period of time. Patients experiencing pain are encouraged to take pain medications one hour before a radiotherapy visit.

It is absolutely essential to remain in exactly the same position during the treatment so the radiation beam is always reaching the exact treatment area, rather than any surrounding tissue. Therapists use molds and other devices to minimize movement and to duplicate the identical position for each treatment.

A therapist will position you under the appropriate machine and then leave the room for the few minutes the machine is on. Because therapists work with radiation

Radiotherapy treatments are very similar to having x-rays. Just as you are not able to see, feel, or hear the rays in a chest x-ray, there is no pain or discomfort with the actual radiation treatment.

every day, it is essential that they leave the room during treatments to avoid getting too much exposure to radiation. The therapist does, however, stay nearby to monitor via television and can communicate with you through a microphone in the treatment room.

52. How long does each treatment take?

Treatments usually take about ten minutes each day. The machine is on for only about one minute for each treatment field; most people have at least two fields. Patients can also expect some waiting time before their actual treatment. The treatment time may be longer if: 1) patients are treated on two different machines or have many fields, or 2) patients have a large field or a complicated set-up.

53. Are there advances in radiation therapy that I should know about?

Advances in radiation technology are allowing more effective treatment of tumors while decreasing the incidence of side effects. **Three-dimensional conformal radiation therapy (3D-CRT)** is a technology that enables doctors to deliver higher doses of radiation to the lung tumor more precisely by using a CT scanner to provide a more accurate measurement of the tumor and its location. Thus, effective doses of radiation can be administered to tumors with less damage to normal tissue. A new type of 3D-CRT technology called **intensity modulated radiation therapy (IMRT)** is currently under investigation. IMRT promises to further increase the effectiveness of radiation treatment by using radiation beams of varying strengths. Tumors are irregular in thickness and shape, and IMRT technology can control the intensity of radiation delivered to different

Three-dimensional conformal radiation therapy (3D-CRT)

A type of radiation therapy that enables higher doses of radiation to be delivered more precisely than standard radiation therapy.

Intensity Modulated Radiation Therapy (IMRT)

A type of three-dimensional radiation therapy (3D-CRT) that uses radiation beams of varying strengths.

Advances in radiation technology are allowing more effective treatment of tumors while decreasing the incidence of side effects.

parts of the tumor, thereby increasing tumor kill and decreasing radiation-induced side effects. **Stereotactic body radiotherapy** is another high-precision technology under investigation for treatment of lung tumors.

Your radiation oncologist can tell you whether any of these technologies might be appropriate treatment options for you.

54. What are the common side effects of radiation therapy?

To get to the tumor, the beam of radiation has to pass through all the tissues in front of and behind the tumor, thereby generating side effects in these normal tissues. For example, radiation to a tumor in the chest must pass in through the skin, the normal lung, the tumor, and then go out through normal lung behind the tumor and the skin. If the tumor is near the esophagus (or "feeding tube") or spinal cord it might pass through a portion of these as well. Because of these side effects, radiation cannot be administered to the entire body; instead, it must be limited to the areas of tumor. The amount of radiation that any one area of the body can tolerate varies. Normal tissues that are extremely sensitive to the effects of radiation, and thus don't tolerate it well include organs within the abdomen and the spinal cord.

The side effects of radiation relate to the amount and nature of normal tissues through which the beam of radiation must pass, as well as to the total dose of radiation given. Therefore, side effects will vary from patient to patient depending upon each patient's treatment plan. In general, however, common side effects of "high dose" (60 Gy, or 6000 rads) radiation on various body tissues are as follows:

Stereotactic body radiotherapy

A highly precise radiation therapy technique; when used to treat brain metastases, it is called stereotactic radiosurgery.

- *Skin.* Radiation side effects to the skin can include a sunburn-like rash. For lung cancer patients, this is rarely a major problem.

- *Normal lungs.* Radiation can cause irritation of the lungs (**pneumonitis**), which can result in shortness of breath and cough. In some patients, this can result in permanent scarring of the lungs (**fibrosis**). Although these side effects are mild and well tolerated in most patients, in some patients with underlying poor lung function, the loss of breath is so significant that the patient may end up on oxygen permanently. Sometimes, the radiotherapist will prescribe steroids if he or she thinks radiation pneumonitis or fibrosis is the cause of the breathing problem.

- *Esophagus.* The esophagus is the tube through which food travels from the mouth to the stomach. Because it passes through the very center of the chest, it often gets exposed to radiation and can become irritated. Irritation of the esophagus usually feels like a sore throat which can sometimes be so bad that patients have a hard time swallowing solid foods. This is a temporary side effect that usually occurs three to four weeks into the radiation treatment, and continues for about two weeks afterward. Rarely, this irritation may cause scarring of the esophagus, which can result in problems with food getting "stuck." If this happens, the patient may need an upper endoscopy, in which a gastroenterologist looks down into the esophagus with a fiberoptic tube or an endoscope, and then uses a balloon at the end of the endoscope to squeeze open the scar tissue and dilate the esophagus.

Pneumonitis
Irritation of the lungs.

Fibrosis
Scarring of the lung.

If the sore throat experienced during radiation therapy becomes too bad, many radiation therapists prescribe a liquid medication containing some lidocaine. Lidocaine can numb the throat, making it easier to eat. During this period of time, do not worry about eating a balanced meal, meat, or solids. It is more important to stay hydrated and consume as many calories as you can, usually in the form of high-protein or calorie shakes, puddings, creamed soups, and the like.

Recent studies in NSCLC patients undergoing chemoradiation treatment found that the drug amifostine (Ethyol) may reduce treatment-related esophageal symptoms. Ask your doctor if a **radioprotectant**, such as amifostine, is available to you.

Radioprotectant
A medication which reduces certain side effects of radiation.

- *Heart.* It is rare to experience heart problems from radiation. The radiotherapist is usually able to direct the beam of radiation so that only small areas of the heart are exposed.

- *Spine.* The spinal cord is very sensitive to radiation and therefore cannot tolerate high doses. Indeed, this is often a factor that limits the amount of radiation that can be delivered, because side effects from spinal radiation are usually permanent. Irritation of the spinal cord can cause back pain and, rarely, numbness, tingling, and weakness of one of the legs, which, in extremely rare cases, can lead to paralysis.

- *Fatigue.* Fatigue is one of the most common side effects of radiation therapy. It is important that you get enough rest during this period. While fatigue can last from 6 weeks to 12 months after your last radiation treatment, it usually gets better one to two weeks after the treatment is finished.

COMBINED MODALITY THERAPY

55. What is combined modality therapy for lung cancer? What are the advantages and disadvantages of this approach?

Combined modality therapy usually means receiving two or more types of treatment: a local treatment (such as radiotherapy or surgery) and systemic chemotherapy. This is usually recommended when a patient has Stage II or locally advanced (Stage III) disease. Combined modality therapy is recommended because such patients often have a high chance of recurrence—either locally (at the site of the original tumor) or distantly (somewhere else in the body). In the latter case, if the cancer comes back somewhere else in the body, it is not the fault of the surgeon—presumably some cancer cells must have spread (metastasized) before the operation. A local recurrence also does not mean that the surgeon did not do his or her job—it means that microscopic amounts of cancer cells, too small for the surgeon to see, were left behind. Therefore, two types of treatment are needed: therapy aimed at the tumor itself (surgery or radiation) and therapy aimed at cancer cells that might have already escaped (chemotherapy or targeted therapy).

The subject of combined modality treatment, and how to administer it, is one of the biggest areas of controversy among lung oncologists.

The subject of combined modality treatment, and how to administer it, is one of the biggest areas of controversy among lung oncologists. When should the doctor give the chemo? Before radiation or surgery? After? Which type of "local" treatment should you have—radiation or surgery? Both? Should the chemotherapy be given at the same time as the radiation? Which chemotherapy is best? Because medical knowledge regarding combination therapy is evolving, you should discuss the pros and cons of each of these approaches with your doctor.

One of the potential disadvantages of combined modality therapy is enhanced side effects.

- If high-dose radiation (60 Gy, or 6000 rads) is given before surgery, the normal tissues become so affected that the body has a hard time healing, and patients can have problems with wounds breaking apart inside the chest. Lower doses of radiation (45 Gy, or 4500 rads) are better tolerated pre-operatively.

- Chemotherapy given concurrently (at the same time) with radiation instead of sequentially (one after the other), in particular, can have more side effects. Patients tend to experience many more problems with fatigue, sore throat, and swallowing. In addition, they are more likely to suffer from radiation pneumonitis and fibrosis (see Question 54). Nevertheless, because there is a survival advantage when the treatment is given this way, it is often recommended, particularly for patients with good performance status (see Question 33).

PART SIX

How will my doctor decide which treatment is best for me?

What are the standard treatment options
for my stage NSCLC?

What are the standard treatment options
for my stage SCLC?

I have SCLC and my doctor has recommended
prophylactic cranial irradiation (PCI).
What is PCI, and how do I decide whether
it is right for me?

More . . .

TREATMENT OF NSCLC

56. What are the standard treatment options for my stage NSCLC?

The standard treatment of NSCLC depends upon several factors, including the stage of the disease and the patient's general health. The first of these will determine which treatment will be recommended; the second will determine whether the treatment needs to be changed in some way.

Please note that the following treatment recommendations are generalizations only. You must talk to your oncologist about your specific case. He or she may change these recommendations based upon the specific circumstances of your situation or your underlying health. In addition, advances in the treatment of lung cancer are being made every day; what is recommended today (or in this book) will almost certainly be outdated tomorrow. An excellent source for current information on lung cancer treatment is the NCI/PDQ Treatment Summaries, which can be found on the National Cancer Institute's web site, *www.cancer.gov*, or the website of the American Society of Clinical Oncology, *www.cancer.net*.

Stages I & II NSCLC

Stage I NSCLC is a tumor that is usually relatively small (less than 3 centimeters, or 1½ inches) and does not involve any lymph nodes. The standard therapy for Stage I NSCLC is surgery, preferably a lobectomy if the patient's underlying lung function is okay, and a wedge resection if it is not. With surgery, the chances of being cured of this cancer run between 60–80%. Some patients, however, cannot tolerate even a wedge resection because their lung function is so poor; other patients may have such significant heart disease that they cannot tolerate any operation. In these cases, high dose radiation can sometimes be given, although it is less likely to be curative compared to surgery.

Stage II NSCLC is a tumor that has spread to the local lymph nodes (also called hilar nodes, or N1 nodes) OR a tumor that is growing into the chest wall, but does not have any lymph node involvement. In both cases, surgery is recommended.

Despite the fact that the tumor has been successfully removed, there is a chance it may come back, either in the lung, or elsewhere (see Question 69). **Adjuvant chemotherapy** is chemotherapy given after surgery, and it has been shown to reduce the chance of lung cancer coming back after lung surgery for patients with Stage II disease, and some patients with Stage I disease who have very large tumors. This is a relatively new finding and some doctors may not be aware of it, so if you have had surgery for Stage I or Stage II lung cancer, be sure to ask your doctor whether you might need adjuvant chemotherapy.

Areas of Research/Clinical Trials (see also Questions 59 and 60)

Although most patients with Stage I lung cancer are cured of their disease, many are not. Lung cancer doctors are exploring several major areas of research for early stage (Stage I and II) patients:

- Can a **chemopreventive agent** prevent the development of lung cancer? In addition to their risk of recurrent disease, patients who develop one lung cancer are at higher risk of developing a second. This risk exists primarily for smokers or former smokers,

Adjuvant therapy

Therapy given after initial treatment to increase its effectiveness; for example, adjuvant chemotherapy following surgery.

Chemopreventive agent

A natural or synthetic substance used to prevent cancer.

Chemoprevention

The use of natural or synthetic substances to prevent cancer.

Neoadjuvant therapy

Therapy given before the primary therapy; for example, neoadjuvant chemotherapy, which is sometimes given prior to surgery.

Radiofrequency ablation (RFA)

Treatment that uses high-frequency electric current to kill cancer cells.

because the carcinogens in tobacco smoke are inhaled into both lungs and may have caused mutations in more than one place. **Chemoprevention** refers to the use of a substance, such as a drug or vitamin, to prevent cancer. There are several large clinical trials looking at the possible role of certain drugs as chemopreventive agents.

- Is neoadjuvant chemotherapy helpful? **Neoadjuvant chemotherapy** is a term for chemotherapy that is given before surgery to kill any microscopic cancer cells that may have already spread, or metastasized, elsewhere in the body. It is given prior to surgery because patients are likely to be stronger and better able to tolerate it, and to attack the microscopic metastases while they are still small.

- What is the role of **radiofrequency ablation (RFA)**? RFA uses high-frequency electric current to kill cancer cells, and some people feel that it can be used instead of surgery. However, this has never been proven; we do not know how it compares to surgery.

- Radiation. Stereotactic body radiotherapy (SBRT) and three-dimensional conformal radiation therapy (3D-CRT), including intensity modulated radiation therapy (IMRT), are all different methods of administering high doses of radiation that are more precise than traditional radiotherapy (see Question 48). Research is underway to determine if administering higher doses with fewer side effects will increase the effectiveness of these radiation techniques in the treatment of lung tumors.

Stage III NSCLC

Stage III NSCLC is a cancer that is big, bulky, and difficult or impossible to resect, but has no obvious signs of metastatic spread. It is typically subdivided into two sub-stages: Stage IIIA, which usually refers to a tumor that is technically operable from a surgeon's viewpoint, and Stage IIIB, which is not. Because the cancer is so large, and that it has spread to mediastinal lymph nodes, the chance that it has already escaped and gone into the blood stream or lymphatics is high. Thus, whether or not to undergo surgery for Stage IIIA is somewhat controversial; many doctors feel high doses of radiation treatment, not surgery, is the best local treatment. Regardless, however, the chances that the cancer has spread are so high that chemotherapy is almost always used as well.

Stage IIIA

Common examples of Stage IIIA disease include:

- Mediastinal lymph node involvement (N2 disease)
- A tumor that is growing into the chest wall and has lymph node involvement (either hilar or mediastinal)

Stage IIIA disease is one disease stage for which combined modality therapy has definitely been shown to improve survival over single agent therapy alone. Again, clinical trials are ongoing to determine which of the following options is best:

- Preoperative (neoadjuvant) chemotherapy followed by surgery
- Preoperative chemotherapy and radiation therapy followed by surgery
- Surgery followed by post-operative (adjuvant) chemotherapy
- Chemotherapy followed by radiation, or radiation followed by chemotherapy
- Chemotherapy given at the same time (concurrently) as radiation therapy

Stage IIIA disease is one disease stage for which combined modality therapy has definitely been shown to improve survival over single agent therapy alone.

Stage IIIB

Common examples of Stage IIIB disease are:

- A tumor that is growing into the heart, trachea, or one of the large vessels leading into or out of the heart
- A tumor with mediastinal lymph nodes on the other side
- Patients with a pleural effusion

In all of these cases, the surgeon cannot completely resect the entire tumor. If all of the tumor cannot be completely resected, surgery is generally NOT recommended. Surgery can be painful, may have side effects or complications, and is rarely curative in this situation. Therefore, it is generally thought that it is not helpful to operate on a patient's tumor unless you can "get it all." In addition, incision lines that contain a few microscopic left over tumor cells have a very hard time healing, so these patients are at increased risk for post-operative complications.

Treatment of Stage IIIB disease usually involves chemotherapy and radiation therapy, except in the case of those patients who have a pleural effusion (see Question 84) from the cancer. In these patients, the cancer cells probably involve the inside of the entire chest wall, which is too large an area to radiate. Therefore, patients with Stage IIIB disease with a pleural effusion generally receive chemotherapy alone, similar to patients with Stage IV disease.

Although it differs depending upon the regimen, most regimens are given about every 3 weeks (a **cycle**). Treatment usually consists of 4–6 cycles, although there is some data to suggest that more cycles may be helpful. For patients with IIIA or IIIB disease without a pleural effusion, most studies show that it is more effective to

Cycle

The schedule of administration of chemotherapy which is repeated 4–6 times.

give the chemotherapy and radiation therapy at the same time ("concurrent" chemo/rads) rather than one after the other (sequentially), even though it has side effects.

Areas of Research/Clinical Trials (see also Questions 59–60)

The treatment of Stage IIIB disease is a very active area of research. Questions that are being explored include:

- Should patients receive additional chemotherapy either before or after the concurrent chemo/rads?
- If the chemo is given at the same time as the radiation, should it be given in standard doses (i.e., high doses every three weeks) or weekly, at lower doses? Should both high dose chemotherapy and weekly low dose chemo with radiotherapy be given, and if so, in what order? What are the best chemotherapy drugs for this situation?
- For those patients who have completed their chemo-radiotherapy, and in whom the tumor appears to have stopped growing, is there anything else that can be given afterward to prevent it from growing?

Stage IV NSCLC

Roughly half of all lung cancer patients will be diagnosed with either Stage IV (metastatic disease) or Stage IIIB with pleural effusion. Unfortunately, at this time, the prospects for cure from Stage IIIB or IV lung cancer are not good. Therefore, the goals of treatment are to prevent the cancer from growing for as long as possible and reduce symptoms and, in doing so, improve both quality of life and survival. Because the cancer has spread, a local therapy is usually not recommended, unless it is to reduce specific symptoms (such as radiotherapy given to help with a painful bony metastasis).

Generally speaking, chemotherapy for patients with Stage IIIB with a pleural effusion or Stage IV NSCLC usually involves a combination of two drugs (a regimen). In the past, one of the two drugs has been a "platin," such as cisplatin or carboplatin, although this does not necessarily have to be the case. The different two-drug regimens differ in how frequently they are given (the **schedule**), how much they cost, and their side effects. In the past, most regimens were about the same in terms of effectiveness; however, it may be that some of the newer drugs will be more effective.

Chemotherapy regimens are given on a regular schedule called a **cycle**. Most (but not all) cycles are every three weeks. For example, a typical three-week cycle involves giving the drug on *Day 1*, and then coming back on *Day 21* for the next cycle. Some drugs may be given more than once during a cycle. Gematabine, for example, is given on days 1 and 8 of a 21-day cycle. The vast majority of regimens are given as an out-patient.

Typically, patients receive 2–3 cycles of chemotherapy and then have a CT scan to determine if the chemotherapy is "working." Remember—doctors are happy if the tumor is the same size or smaller, as long as it is not bigger. If the cancer is **stable** (e.g. the same size) or **responding** (smaller), the doctor will give another 2–3 cycles and again repeat the scan. The doctor usually stops after 4–6 cycles, because most studies have shown that more is not helpful, and the side effects, particularly fatigue and myelosuppression, tend to catch up with a person.

Avastin ("bevacizumab") is often given in combination with chemotherapy to patients who do not have squamous cell carcinoma and are not at risk for other complications (ask your doctor). There is some data to

Schedule

How frequently chemotherapy is given.

Cycle

The schedule of administration of chemotherapy which is repeated 4–6 times.

Typically, patients receive 2–3 cycles of chemotherapy and then have a CT scan to determine if the chemotherapy is "working."

Stable disease

Cancer which has stopped growing following treatment.

Responding disease

Cancer which has shrunk in response to chemotherapy.

suggest that Erbitux (cetuximab) may also be helpful, although at the time of this writing, it has not yet been approved for NSCLC.

A number of different chemotherapy regimens are used for the treatment of advanced NSCLC. (see Table 3) They differ in terms of their side effects, cost, and how frequently they are given. It is beyond the scope of this book to discuss the pros and cons of each. Indeed, by the time this book is published, almost certainly more will have been approved. You should have a frank discussion with your medical oncologist regarding the pros and cons of the different regimens.

Areas of Research/Clinical Trials (see also Questions 59 and 60)

Targeted therapy is an active area of research for treatment of metastatic NSCLC. Scientists are making considerable advances in learning the many different ways cancer cells differ from normal cells, and as they do so, they are making new drugs to target these differences.

TREATMENT OF SCLC

57. What are the standard treatment options for my stage SCLC?

Limited Stage

Limited Stage SCLC is potentially a curable disease. The optimal treatment consists of chemotherapy (usually four cycles) plus concurrent radiation therapy to the chest. However, as discussed in Question 55, this combination has significant side effects and probably should not be given to patients who are frail or who have bad lungs. Some physicians try to minimize the toxicity by giving the chemotherapy and radiation therapy sequentially instead of concurrently. In limited stage SCLC, this is probably not as helpful as giving them at the same time. At least one study showed that if the radiation therapy is given twice per day for 12–15 days instead of once per day for 20–25 fractions, patients are more likely to be cured.

Areas of Research/Clinical Trials (see also Questions 59 and 60)

Active areas of investigation include:
- What is the best dose of radiation therapy, and how frequently should it be delivered?
- What is the best chemotherapy?
- Are there any other treatments that can be administered after the chemotherapy is done to prevent the cancer from coming back?

Extensive Stage SCLC

The principles behind chemotherapy for SCLC are the same as for NSCLC. Although patients with advanced, metastatic SCLC are rarely cured, they very often respond to chemotherapy, at least for a while. The typical chemotherapy regimens in the past have been a platin (carboplatin or cisplatin) plus etoposide (VP-16).

Areas of Research/Clinical Trials (see also Questions 59 and 60)

An active area of clinical investigation is trying to identify types of chemotherapy regimens.

58. I have SCLC and my doctor has recommended prophylactic cranial irradiation (PCI). What is PCI, and how do I decide whether it is right for me?

Prophylactic cranial irradiation (PCI) is radiation to the brain with the intention of preventing the development of brain metastases. It is based on the premise that chemotherapy does not penetrate well into the brain, so there may be micrometastases in the brain that have not been exposed to chemotherapy. PCI is recommended for SCLC patients who achieve complete **remission** following initial treatment because the brain is a common site of recurrence for SCLC. PCI reduces the incidence of brain metastases and improves both disease-free and overall survival for SCLC patients in complete remission.

The potential for mental impairment remains a primary concern for patients considering PCI. For most patients, this concern is unfounded. Although further research is needed, two large studies have shown that the long-term consequences of PCI on mental functioning are slight. The primary side effect of PCI is reversible hair loss.

If you are a candidate for PCI, you should discuss its pros and cons with both your oncologist and your radiation oncologist. An important question to ask is whether there is anything about you as an individual that puts you at risk for side effects. Although the risks from PCI are limited, certain patients may be more susceptible to side effects. Because SCLC patients face a high prospect of brain metastases—which are associated with disabling symptoms and early death—the decision to undergo PCI makes sense in most cases when considering both quality of life and survival.

Prophylactic cranial irradiation (PCI)

Radiation to the brain with the intention of preventing the development of brain metastases.

Remission

Shrinkage of tumor in response to treatment. May be either "complete" (total disappearance of tumor) or partial (the tumor has shrunk, but has not gone away entirely).

INVESTIGATIVE/EXPERIMENTAL THERAPIES

59. What are clinical trials?

Clinical trials are research studies involving people (as opposed to preclinical studies which may involve animals). Through clinical trials, scientists learn how to fight cancer. There are many types of clinical trials (prevention, screening, treatment, quality-of-life) and questions that scientists can address by means of a clinical trial. The clinical trials process is designed to encourage the development of new drugs for cancer while protecting the volunteers who participate in the trials.

The clinical trials process is designed to encourage the development of new drugs for cancer while protecting the volunteers who participate in the trials.

Participating in a clinical trial may sound scary. However, this is the only way any progress is made in the treatment of cancer. All drugs that we now have to treat cancer were developed through clinical trials, in which patients such as you participated. There are many reasons for participating in a clinical trial, but even if you do not benefit directly, the knowledge gained from your participation will help future lung cancer patients. The clinical trials process for a new cancer drug begins with an application by the study sponsor to the Food and Drug Administration (FDA) to conduct a clinical trial. The FDA is the U.S. government agency that approves new treatments for marketing and sale to the public. It provides oversight and approval for new drugs, new devices, new types of treatments, and new uses for established drugs, devices, and treatments. For most cancer trials, the study sponsor is either the National Cancer Institute (or one of its associated trial groups, including the Eastern Cooperative Oncology Group [ECOG], the Southwestern Cooperative Oncology Group [SWOG], the American College of Surgeons Oncology Group [ACOSOG], the Cancer and Leukemia Group B [CALGB]), or a drug company. The study sponsor must demonstrate that testing of the drug in laboratory studies ("in vitro" studies, meaning in a Petrie dish or flask) and in animal studies ("in vivo" studies) showed promise with a reasonable expectation of safety in humans. After the investigational new drug (IND) application is approved, an investigational drug will usually undergo three phases of testing, before it is eligible for final FDA approval:

- Phase I trials are designed to test the *safety* of the new drug. They usually involve a small number of patients (usually fewer than 50) who are given the drug in gradually increasing amounts to assess side effects and establish the most appropriate dose and schedule.

- Phase II trials determine how *effective* the drug is for treating a specific cancer. Phase II trials are usually conducted in larger groups of people (anywhere from 25 to 200). If the drug looks like it might have activity in a certain tumor type, then a Phase III trial is conducted.

- Phase III trials are designed to test whether a new drug is better than the standard treatment for a specific cancer. Both the effectiveness of the drug and the amount and extent of side effects are compared. The number of people participating in Phase III trials can range from hundreds to thousands, and typically involve dozens of hospitals in the United States, and sometimes world-wide.

Phase III trials frequently employ a trial design called a **randomized controlled trial (RCT)**. In a RCT, the trial participants are randomly assigned (by chance, like the flip of a coin, although the randomization process is usually performed by a computer) to the treatment (experimental) group or the control (standard of care) group. You

Randomized controlled trial (RCT)

A research study in which the participants are assigned by chance (using a computer or a table of random numbers) to separate groups that compare different treatments; a method used to prevent bias in research.

Arms of a clinical study

Treatment group to which a patient is assigned in a RTC.

may hear these groups referred to as **arms**. The experimental arm receives the new treatment alone, or the new treatment combined with standard treatment. The control arm receives the standard treatment. Assignment to one arm or another is not based on any medical information; it is "random." Some trials are double-blinded, which means that neither the patients nor the doctors know who is in the experimental group and who is in the control group.

Randomization, control, and blinding are all scientific methods used to ensure that the trial results will not be biased in favor of one outcome or another. If clinical trials were not randomized, physicians might tend to refer all of one type of patient or another to a particular arm of the study. For example, if the medical oncologist thinks a drug is particularly promising but is worried about side effects, given the option, he or she might decide to enter only the youngest patients into the investigational arm of the study, and enter the older patients into the control arm, thereby possibly biasing the results.

Placebo

An inactive substance (e.g., sugar pill). Placebos are rarely used in cancer trials.

One type of trial design that concerns many patients is a **placebo**-controlled trial. A placebo is a dummy or inactive substance (like a sugar pill) that is given to individuals in the control arm of certain trials. Some cancer patients avoid clinical trials for fear of getting a placebo. This fear is unfounded. *It is extremely rare that a placebo-only arm is used in a cancer treatment trial.* It is unethical to treat patients with a placebo when effective care is available, even if it is in the context of testing a promising new drug. The only circumstances in which a placebo-only arm is used in a treatment trial is if the standard of care for that type and stage of cancer is no treatment at all, or in a RCT in which the two arms are "standard chemo + study drug," or "standard chemo + placebo." In either case, both arms get standard chemo. Your doctor will tell you if a study involves a placebo, but you should ask in any case.

60. How do I learn about clinical trials? How do I evaluate whether a trial is the right one for me?

Your first step should be to ask your oncologist whether a clinical trial might be appropriate for you. He or she may recommend a specific trial or trials and can discuss the pros and cons of your participation. You may also want to research clinical trials yourself to increase the chances that you have covered all of your options. (This task can be delegated to a family member or friend if you are not up to the effort.) Your oncologist will be able to help you evaluate what you find. (For information on how to locate clinical trials, see the clinical trials locators listed in Appendix A.)

Before a study can begin, it must be reviewed by the Institutional Review Board (IRB) to make sure that the study is ethical (e.g., patients are not being denied an effective treatment), and as safe as possible. The IRB is an independent committee of the hospital which makes sure that clinical studies meet ethical guidelines, and that prospective participants are given all the information they need in order to make an **informed consent**.

If your doctor does not have access to clinical trials, the next step is to contact the principal investigator, or study coordinator, of the trial itself. He or she will evaluate your eligibility for the trial by reviewing the inclusion criteria (for example, type and stage of lung cancer) and exclusion criteria (for example, some studies might exclude patients with kidney disease for safety reasons

Informed consent

A process that provides potential participants in a clinical trial the information they need to make an informed decision about whether or not to participate.

or require potential participants to have had no prior chemotherapy). Eligibility criteria are used to protect participants and also to ensure that the study participants are alike in certain ways so that trial results will be more reliable.

Before you sign the informed consent document, ask your doctor who will cover the costs of the trial, including the costs of treating any unexpected side effects. Be sure you understand everything and that you discuss it with whomever you trust to help you with your medical decisions.

After it has been determined that you are a potential candidate for the trial, the informed consent process begins. The process of informed consent is designed to protect your interests and safety as a trial participant in a scientific experiment by giving you the information you need to make an informed decision about whether to participate. The process begins when the investigator or study coordinator explains the trial to you. He or she will describe the purpose of the study, why you are eligible, how many people are participating, the procedures and design of the trial, the anticipated risks (which may include physical, financial, psychological, and legal risks in addition to any potential risks to your privacy/confidentiality), the costs of the trial, if any, as well as alternatives that may be open to you other than the trial. Your rights as a trial participant should be made clear: that your participation in a clinical trial is voluntary, that you are free to stop the study at any time, and that there will be no penalty if you decide to stop (e.g., Your doctor will not be angry at you). Before you sign the informed consent document, ask your doctor who will cover the costs of the trial, including the costs of treating any unexpected side effects. Be sure you understand everything and that you discuss it with whomever you trust to help you with your medical decisions.

There are many good reasons why you might consider participating in a clinical trial: you may have run out of the standard treatments available to treat your lung cancer; you may feel that standard therapies don't have much to offer you and that a potential new drug holds more promise; you may feel that you will get better care in a clinical trial; or you may want to help patients who come after you. Whatever your motive(s), you should be sure you understand the differences (in terms of risks, benefits, and practical considerations, such as time and cost) between a clinical trial and your other options. Only then can you make a truly informed decision.

ALTERNATIVE THERAPIES

61. What is alternative medicine?

Alternative medicine generally refers to therapies developed outside of mainstream medicine and used in place of standard, clinically proven therapies. Some of these therapies are touted as "cures" for cancer, with little or no scientific information to support them. It is often impossible to establish the reliability of individual testimonials, locate scientific research on alternative therapies, or verify the credentials of an alternative medicine practitioner. Unproved alternative therapies are often promoted and sold by the same person, a charlatan who attempts to take advantage of vulnerable cancer patients. Insurance does not cover these types of alternative treatments. The cost of alternative medicine can be significant in terms of dollars, and in wasted time and energy. Most importantly, they can be dangerous to your health.

On the other hand, "alternative medicine" can also describe traditional medical systems, such as Traditional Chinese Medicine (TCM) or Ayurveda (from India). Although these systems have been in use for centuries, they have not been studied with the same scientific rigor as Western medicine. Because of this lack of data, many in the Western medical community view these alternative systems with skepticism and resistance.

When alternative methods are used in addition to conventional therapy, it is often referred to as complementary medicine. Although complementary medicine can include approaches such as herbal therapies, the term often refers to methods such as acupuncture and mind/body techniques (guided imagery, meditation) that are aimed at improving side effects and symptoms rather than curing disease. Complementary methods can range from nutritional supplements and herbal therapies, to hypnotism and biofeedback, to art therapy and spiritual practices.

There has long been a disconnect between patients and doctors with regard to the use of complementary and alternative medicine (CAM). A significant percentage of patients use some type of complementary therapy but do not share this information with their doctors. Some patients feel that their doctors would not be receptive; others see no reason to tell their doctors. Doctors often fail to ask patients about their use of complementary medicine. For some doctors this may reflect a bias against alternative methods or a lack of expertise; for others it may reflect an ignorance or lack of concern about the prevalence of CAM use among patients. Poor communication on CAM issues may compromise patient care. The good news is that there is more ongoing scientific research into CAM therapies, thereby encouraging awareness and dialogue on CAM issues. The National Institute of Health has established the National Center for Complementary and Alternative Medicine (NCCAM), dedicated to encouraging research and distributing accurate information on CAM therapies. The National Cancer Institute's Office of Cancer Complementary and Alternative Medicine (OCCAM) supports the NCCAM mandate, focusing specifically on CAM for cancer.

- If you are interested in pursuing alternative thera-pies, first check the NCCAM (*www.nccam.nih.gov*) and OCCAM (*www.cancer.gov/cam/*) web sites to see if there is evidence of safety and effectiveness. This should be done for both alternative and comple-mentary treatments. You will find comprehensive fact sheets and summaries on individual therapies (e.g., antineoplastons, acupuncture, coenzyme Q10, dietary supplements) with links to both CAM clin-ical trials and CAM scientific literature. Another valuable resource for checking the reliability of alternative therapies marketed to cancer patients is Quackwatch (*www.quackwatch.com*). Quackwatch reviews the evidence and provides critiques of these therapies and should be consulted prior to undergo-ing any alternative treatment. Your doctor can help you to evaluate what you find in your research and advise you on whether a therapy or method might make sense for you.

- It is crucial to understand that herbal treatments and dietary supplements (vitamins) are not regu-lated by the Food and Drug Administration (FDA), and therefore any claims about anti-tumor efficacy have not been proven or reproduced by independent investigators. There are also reasons to be concerned about quality control, as well as issues of safety and effectiveness in these substances that you may con-sider safe. The best policy is to discuss the possible consequences of taking these substances with your doctor before you take them.

- Check the credentials of your CAM practitioner carefully. Ask for information on education, train-ing, and membership in professional organizations. Complementary therapies abound. Some patients find that activities such as meditation, guided imagery, yoga, and tai chi help them to relieve pain, stress, and anxiety, and increase their quality-of-life. There is little scientific data, however, that they are helpful in controlling cancer. For further information on the complementary therapies available to you, check with your hospital's patient center, or contact a cancer support organization such as CancerCare or the Wellness Community.

TREATMENT OF SPECIAL POPULATIONS AND CONDITIONS

62. I am 78 years old. Am I too old for chemo? Will it be too tough on me? Are there particular considerations for treatment of elderly lung cancer patients?

Age alone should not prevent you from receiving treatment for lung cancer.

Age alone should not prevent you from receiving treatment for lung cancer. Elderly patients can undergo chemotherapy, radiation, and/or surgery if their overall health allows them to withstand the stress of treatment. Generally speaking, older patients tolerate treatment as well as their younger counterparts, providing they are healthy. Your doctor will determine your ability to undergo treatment by assessing your level of function (called performance status—see Question 33) and any coexisting medical problems that may complicate some treatments. These circumstances are often a primary consideration when determining treatment options. However, it is important to recognize that your overall condition is a better predictor of your ability to tolerate treatment than is your chronological age.

When a chemotherapy drug is given alone as treatment, it is called monotherapy. Several chemotherapy drugs have been studied for use as monotherapies in elderly lung cancer patients with encouraging outcomes and fewer side effects than the standard multi-drug regimens. These chemotherapies include vinorelbine, docetaxel, Alimta, gemcitabine, and paclitaxel. Although elderly patients with good performance status can undergo standard chemotherapy regimens involving multiple drugs, patients with less-than-optimal performance status are frequently ineligible for regimens involving multiple adverse effects. Single-drug regimens can be a good choice for these patients, offering less toxicity without sacrificing effectiveness. Some of the newer, experimental treatment agents may also be appropriate for patients with poor performance status because many of these agents target tumor cells and leave normal cells unaffected, resulting in fewer and less toxic side effects.

For lobectomy or wedge resections, age alone is not a risk factor, and elderly patients who are otherwise healthy should not be denied these surgical options based on chronological age. When surgery involves removal of the entire lung (pneumonectomy), however, there is a considerable risk of post-op complications and death over the age of 70. Pneumonectomy in the elderly should be undertaken with great caution and consideration. When feasible, video-assisted thoracoscopic surgery (VATS) offers a safer, less invasive alternative to traditional, open procedures for all lung cancer patients. Alternative treatment options are available for patients who are judged to be medically inoperable (due to poor performance status or coexisting illnesses). For example, radiotherapy (with curative intent) has been used in elderly patients who are not surgical candidates, but who have potentially curable early stage NSCLC.

If you are elderly with lung cancer, you should be alert to any age bias on the part of your doctor—it is both inappropriate and substandard care to receive less aggressive treatment solely because of your age. Elderly patients who are in good health and have a good performance status face no greater risks from standard treatments based on their age alone. For those elderly patients with compromised performance status and/or limiting illness, there may be alternative treatment options available. Communication with your doctor is essential to learning all of your treatment options. Only then can you make an informed decision based on what is right for you—whatever your age.

63. Are there specific treatments available for bronchioloalveolar carcinoma (BAC)?

Bronchioloalveolar carcinoma (BAC) is a sub-type of adenocarcinoma, where the cancer tends to spread diffusely throughout the alveoli in the lung (see Question 4). This often gives a somewhat hazy appearance on a chest x-ray, similar to pneumonia, instead of a solid tumor mass. The disease progression of BAC tends to vary somewhat from pure adenocarcinoma—BAC is considered slower growing and less likely to metastasize, although the overall prognosis remains similar to other types of NSCLC. BAC also tends to occur in patients who have never smoked, and in younger women.

Currently, BAC is treated the same as adenocarcinoma and other forms of NSCLC. However, many studies now show that patients with BAC tend to respond better to an EGFR inhibitor, such as Tarceva (see Question 44), than do patients with other types (histologies) of lung cancer. Although it is not yet known if BAC patients respond better to Tarceva than to chemotherapy, this area of research is advancing rapidly, with new discoveries being reported on a frequent basis. If you have BAC, it makes sense to contact one of the clinical investigators on the BAC studies. (See Appendix A for clinical trials locators.) Because BAC is relatively rare, most doctors do not have experience with BAC and cannot advise you on the particular concerns related to BAC. Because doctors who participate on BAC trials tend to see more BAC patients than other doctors, they may be a good resource for you, whether or not you decide to participate in a BAC trial.

64. My doctor told me that I have developed brain metastases. What are my treatment options?

There are several ways to treat brain metastases, and your doctor will advise you about which treatments may be appropriate in your individual case. Traditional surgery may occasionally be used to remove a brain metastasis, particularly if there is only one metastasis and the tumor elsewhere in your body is under relatively good control. More likely, you will be treated with radiation. Whole brain radiation may be used to shrink or eradicate the tumors if you have numerous small metastases. Stereotactic radiosurgery (pinpoint radiation; also known as "Gamma Knife" or "Cyber Knife," depending upon the machine being used) may be used alone or in conjunction with whole brain radiation when there are only a few small metastases. In some cases, chemotherapy used to treat primary brain tumors has been used in patients with brain metastases, but there is no evidence that these treatments are effective in prolonging survival for lung cancer patients.

There are several ways to treat brain metastases, and your doctor will advise you about which treatments may be appropriate in your individual case.

119

65. How are bone metastases treated?

If your lung cancer has metastasized to your bones, treatment will be aimed at reducing pain and strengthening the bone to reduce the risk of fractures. Common sites of bone metastasis are the vertebrae, ribs, hips, leg, and arm bones. Traditional radiation therapy to the involved area is effective for reducing pain. Occasionally, if the tumor has weakened the bone to the verge of breaking, surgery may be recommended to remove the bone tumor and stabilize the bone to prevent future breakage. Another method for treating bone metastases is drug therapy using a class of drugs called bisphosphonates, such as Zometa (zoledronic acid). Given intravenously, Zometa strengthens bone, thus reducing the chance of developing bone metastasis.

EVALUATING TREATMENT OPTIONS AND OUTCOMES

66. How do I decide on a treatment plan when I am faced with multiple options?

This is a difficult question. Talk with your doctor, and make sure you know all of your treatment options and that you understand the differences among them. Carefully weigh the pros and cons of each treatment, and evaluate your priorities. Many factors may influence your decision. These may include treatment survival rates, side effects and quality of life concerns, cost, time commitment, travel, and so on. If, for example, being home as much as possible is one of your top priorities, you would be less likely to choose a daily intravenous treatment than one that requires coming to the hospital only once every three weeks.

Your doctor will advise you on your options and make treatment recommendations based upon his or her medical experience and training and on what he or she knows about you, your tumor, and your priorities. Many patients feel pressured and/or overwhelmed with having to make the decision and prefer to follow their doctor's recommendation. Other people like to be more actively involved in the decision-making process. Whatever your preference, the doctor–patient relationship is a critical component of the process. If you communicate effectively with your doctor regarding what you want from your treatment, it will allow him or her to provide you with optimal treatment advice.

67. How do I know if my treatment is working? What is the difference between partial response and complete response? What is a remission?

A remission is another word for response. For some reason hematologists tend to use the word "remission" for leukemia and lymphoma, while oncologists (solid tumor doctors) tend to use the word response when talking about cancers such as lung cancer. A **partial response** (or **partial remission**) is defined as an approximate 30% shrinkage of the tumor as determined by x-ray, CT scan, or physical exam. A **complete response** (or **complete remission**) is total disappearance of the tumor. Note, however, that neither a partial nor a complete response necessarily translates into "cure." It is not uncommon for a patient to have a temporary response, meaning that the tumor initially shrinks with chemotherapy but then starts

Partial response

A decrease in the size of a tumor, or in the extent of cancer in the body, in response to treatment. Also called **partial remission**.

Complete response

The disappearance of all signs of cancer in response to treatment. This does not always mean the cancer has been cured. Also called **complete remission**.

to grow at some point. Probably, the chemotherapy killed off the "sensitive" cancer cells, leaving behind a population of cancer cells that were more resistant to chemotherapy, and which eventually started to grow.

In the past, the "official" way to tell whether the treatment is working is to get another scan and see whether the tumor is shrinking. Many patients can tell even before the scan is taken, because their symptoms from the cancer improve as the tumor shrinks. However, many chemotherapy regimens don't actually shrink the tumor—they stop it from growing ("stable" disease).

68. What if my disease has remained stable during treatment?

If your disease is stable, that's good! It means you and your doctor are achieving your goal—stopping the cancer from growing. There are many cases in which a patient's tumor never shrank according to a CT scan, but never grew either. Presumably, in these situations the cancer cells must have been killed by the treatment but never disintegrated enough to make it look like the tumor was shrinking. Another possibility is that the tumor on the scan could now contain a lot of scar tissue that formed from the treatment.

69. What happens if my disease recurs? How is recurrence treated? Is it possible to survive a recurrence of lung cancer?

Recurrence is something that every lung cancer patient fears. If you have experienced a recurrence, do not despair. Although cure following a recurrence is rare, long-term survival is not impossible. Try not to let yourself become overwhelmed or paralyzed by this news—it is almost always the case that you will have treatment options that can increase your survival. Discuss these options with your doctor, including clinical trials, of which there are many (see Questions 59 and 60). Follow the same decision-making process as you did when you were initially diagnosed. Weigh the pros and cons of each option. Make informed decisions. When dealing with recurrent lung cancer or lung cancer that does not respond to treatment, it is especially important that you communicate with your doctor regarding your changing needs and priorities.

Ask yourself how aggressive you want to be. Each time the tumor grows after treatment, it tends to become slightly more resistant to chemotherapy. You may find that quality of life becomes a greater concern if your disease continues to progress despite treatment. However, if aggressively attacking the tumor as much as possible is something you want to do, advocate for yourself. Ask your physician very specifically what the alternative treatments are. If he or she cannot provide any, seek a second opinion at an academic cancer center (see Questions 20 and 21).

Chemotherapy Drugs for Lung Cancer

Chemotherapy recommendations vary depending on whether you have NSCLC or SCLC. New types of chemotherapy are under development all the time; this book is not meant to discuss them in detail. (See Part 7 for Side Effects.)

NSCLC

For NSCLC, **first-line therapy** (i.e., initial treatment) will often consist of two drugs, one of which is usually a "platinum" (cisplatin or carboplatin). Available non-platinum drugs include docetaxel (Taxotere),

First-line therapy
Initial treatment.

gemcitabine (Gemzar), paclitaxel (Taxol), pemetrexed (Alimta) and vinorelbine (Navelbine). In general, the two-drug regimens used for NSCLC have roughly the same success rate in shrinking the tumor and prolonging life. However, they do have different side effects, schedules of administration, and cost, so many oncologists will base their decision on which one to recommend based on these factors. Bevacizumab (Avastin) is often added for those patients who do not have squamous cell carcinoma, brain metastases, bleeding or clotting problems, and who have not coughed up any blood (hemoptysis).

Should lung cancer progress during or following initial chemotherapy, oncologists will often recommend additional therapy. Docetaxel (Taxotere) and pemetrexed (Alimta) are two chemotherapy drugs that have been approved in the United States for **second-line treatment** of NSCLC. Oncologists sometimes use gemcitabine (Gemzar) if the patient did not receive it previously. Erlotinib (Tarceva), a targeted therapy, has been approved for both second and third-line treatment. Your oncologist can tell you which option makes sense for your situation.

Second-line treatment

Treatment method(s) used following an initial treatment that either does not stop cancer progression or stops it only temporarily.

SCLC

For SCLC, first-line therapy is often etoposide (VP-16) and either cisplatin or carboplatin. Second-line therapy for SCLC may include the following additional regimens and drugs: cyclophosphamide, doxorubicin, vincristine; carboplatin, etoposide (VP-16) and ifosfamide; and topotecan.

How to Learn More About Chemotherapy Drugs

It is best to discuss your chemotherapy alternatives with your oncologist because new chemotherapy drugs and regimens are constantly under development. Your oncologist will be able to advise you on the likely side effects. If you are interested in further information about chemotherapy drugs, you can consult the following resources:

Clinical Research

To learn more about the effectiveness of lung cancer chemotherapies, you can search the medical literature via PubMed at: *www.pubmed.org*. Enter the term "lung cancer" (use quotes) and the drug name in the search box separated by the word "AND" in all capital letters—for example: "lung cancer" AND carboplatin.

You can further refine your search by clicking on the LIMIT button, which allows you to limit your search in various ways, such as by date, language, and type of publication.

To learn more about the effectiveness of lung cancer chemotherapies, you can search the medical literature via PubMed at: www.pubmed.org.

Side Effects

Ask your oncologist about the potential side effects of your chemotherapy regimen. He or she will be able to tell you what to expect and what to do if you experience side effects. MEDLINEplus, the National Library of Medicine's consumer health web site, is also an excellent source of detailed information on chemotherapies and other drugs. For each drug, MEDLINEplus lists the brand name(s); a description; things to know before using the drug, such as allergy or pregnancy considerations; and a list of common, less common, and rare side effects. To access the MEDLINEplus drug database, go to *www.medlineplus.gov* and click on "Drugs & Supplements." *The Consumers Guide to Cancer Drugs* (by Gail Wilkes, published by Jones and Bartlett Publishers, 2003) provides similar information on chemotherapy drug side effects.

PART SEVEN

Side Effects of Chemotherapy

What are the common side effects of chemotherapy?

What are blood counts, and what should I know about them?

Why am I always exhausted? What can I do for fatigue? Will the fatigue go away after my treatment is over?

More . . .

70. What are the common side effects of chemotherapy?

The particular side effects you experience will depend on which chemotherapy drugs you receive and your individual response. You should ask your oncologist or oncology nurse for information on the common side effects associated with your chemotherapy regimen. You need to be aware of how to manage the common effects and under what circumstances you should call your oncologist. Some patients find it helpful to keep a journal during chemotherapy treatment to record the dates, times, and duration of symptoms, along with descriptive information. The more accurate you can be in reporting your symptoms to your oncologist, the better care you will receive.

The more accurate you can be in reporting your symptoms to your oncologist, the better care you will receive.

Although there are numerous side effects associated with chemotherapy, it is important to remember that no one gets all of them. In fact, most patients experience relatively few side effects. Common chemotherapy side effects include:

- Fatigue. Fatigue is one of the most commons side effects of chemotherapy, although for most patients, it is relatively mild. It tends to be at its worst for about one week following chemotherapy. Many lung cancer patients are able to continue working, although many cut back to part time. If your fatigue is overwhelming, tell your doctor because there may be something else going on.
- Hair loss (alopecia). Please note that not all lung cancer chemotherapy drugs cause hair loss! Ask your doctor! (see Table 3)
- Mild nausea and, rarely, vomiting
- Drop in blood counts (white blood cells, red blood cells or platelets). This is called myelosuppression, and is a potentially serious side effect of chemotherapy. (see Question 71)

Less common effects:

- Infection
- Skin and nail problems
- Loss of appetite
- Peripheral neuropathy
- Allergic reactions
- Sexual effects: desire, fertility, hormonal balance
- Oral effects: sore mouth and gums, changes in taste
- Gastrointestinal effects: diarrhea and constipation

71. What are blood counts, and what should I know about them?

To monitor the effects of chemotherapy on your blood count (hematologic effects), your oncologist will order a test called a complete blood count (CBC). A CBC counts each type of blood cell. Blood tests are usually performed prior to chemo, and may be performed when counts are predicted to be low. Low blood counts may cause your chemotherapy treatments to be postponed or modified until the passage of time brings them back to safe levels. There are also medications your doctor can prescribe.

You should be aware of the following conditions caused by the effect of chemotherapy on blood counts:

Neutropenia: a low white blood cell (WBC) count. White blood cells fight infection in your body. **Neutrophils** are one type of white blood cell that attacks bacteria. If your neutrophil count (called absolute neutrophil count, or ANC) drops to low levels, you are at higher risk of infection, including serious, potentially life-threatening side effects such as pneumonia. **Neutropenia** can be a dangerous condition for

Neutrophil

A type of white blood cell that attacks bacteria.

Neutropenia

Low white blood cell count.

Table 3 Selected side effects of drugs which are commonly used for the treatment of lung cancer*

Drugs which cause myelosuppression (a temporary drop in the blood counts):	Drugs which cause minimal or no myelosuppression:
• Taxol (paclitaxel)	• Cisplatin
• Taxotere (docetaxel)	• Alimta (pemetrexed)
• Cytoxan (cyclophosphamide)	• Avastin (bevacizumab)
• Adriamycin (doxorubicin)	• Tarceva (erlotinib)
• Vespid (etoposide)	• Erbitux (cetuximab)
• Navelbine (vinorelbine)	
• Carboplatin	
• Topotecan	
• Gemzar (gemcitabine)	

Drugs which are likely to cause almost complete hair loss:	Drugs which cause mild to moderate hair loss:	Drugs which cause only mild or no hair loss:
• Taxol (paclitaxel)	• Vespid (etoposide)	• Cisplatin
• Taxotere (docetaxel)	• Navelbine (vinorelbine)	• Gemzar (gemcitabine)
• Cytoxan (cyclophosphamide)	• Carboplatin	• Alimta (pemetrexed)
• Adriamycin (doxorubicin)	• Topotecan	• Avastin (bevacizumab)
		• Tarceva (erlotinib)
		• Erbitux (cetuximab)

Drugs which can cause nausea, unless the proper anti-emetics are given:	Drugs which can cause mild nausea (usually well controlled by anti-emetics):	Drugs which generally cause minimal nausea:
• Cisplatin	• Taxol (paclitaxel)	• Alimta (pemetrexed)
	• Taxotere (docetaxel)	• Avastin (Bevacizumab)
	• Carboplatin	• Tarceva (erlotinib)
	• Gemzar (gemcitabine)	• Erbitux (cetuximab)

Drugs which can cause allergic reactions:
- Taxol (paclitaxel)
- Taxotere (docetaxel)
- Erbitux (cetuximab)
- Cytoxan (cyclophosphamide)

Drugs which can cause numbness and tingling in the hands and feet (peripheral neuropathy)
- Taxol (paclitaxel)
- Taxotere (docetaxel)
- Cisplatin

Drugs which can cause skin rash:
- Tarceva (erlotinib)
- Erbitux (cetuximab)

Drugs which can cause hypertension:
- Avastin (bevacizumab)

* Please note that this is not a comprehensive list. Also, it does not include drugs which are used for the treatment of other types of cancer. Talk to your doctor about which drugs are best for you.

a cancer patient because infections in neutrapenic patients tend to be more severe than in other individuals and may require hospitalization for IV antibiotics. If your counts indicate that your neutrophils are significantly below normal (a period called the **nadir** that usually occurs 10–14 days following treatment), you should avoid situations that might increase your risk of infection. For example, you can wash your hands frequently, avoid crowds (shopping malls, movie theaters, classrooms) or exposure to individuals with illness, and avoid eating uncooked and undercooked foods. Neutropenia can be treated with drugs called **colony-stimulating factors** (such as Neupogen, Neulasta, and Leukine) that cause your bone marrow to increase the number of white blood cells. If you experience fever, chills, sweats, or other symptoms of infection while getting chemo, you should contact your oncologist's office promptly.

Although neutropenia can occur with almost all types of chemotherapy, the chemotherapy commonly used in lung cancer does not usually result in neutropenia that is so severe, or of such a long duration, that patients come down with an infection. Fortunately, the chances of coming down with an infection is relatively low for lung cancer patients compared to other cancer patients, who get different types of chemotherapy.

Anemia: a low **red blood cell** (**RBC**) count. Your red blood cells carry oxygen to your body. A low RBC count means that there is not enough oxygen in your blood—you are anemic. Your oncologist may refer to a low **hematocrit** (a measure of the number of RBCs in your blood) or a low **hemoglobin** (a protein in RBCs), two specific measures for anemia. If you become anemic, you may experience fatigue,

SIDE EFFECTS OF CHEMOTHERAPY

Nadir
Lowest measured value; period of low blood counts.

Colony-stimulating factors
Substances that stimulate bone marrow to increase production of blood cells; also referred to as hematologic growth factors.

Anemia
Low red blood cell count; may cause tiredness, weakness, and shortness of breath.

Red blood cell
The most common type of blood cell and the vertebrate body's principal means of delivering oxygen to the body tissues via the blood.

Hematocrit
The proportion of the blood that consists of packed red blood cells.

Hemoglobin
The oxygen-carrying protein pigment in the blood, specifically in the red blood cells.

weakness, and dizziness; headache and shortness of breath can also be symptoms of anemia. In some cases, a blood transfusion may be necessary to restore your RBC count to safe levels. In the past, physicians often gave a medication called erythropoetin (Epo; ProCrit; Aranesp) to increase the number of RBCs. However, these medications have become very controversial, since they have recently been found to cause blood clots, and in some cancers, increase the risk of death. Because of this, at the time of this writing, the FDA is considering significantly restricting the use of these medications in cancer patients.

Thrombocytopenia: low platelet levels. Platelets are a type of blood cell which helps stop bleeding. Patients with low levels of platelets may experience bruising or bleeding (e.g., nosebleeds, bleeding gums, intestinal bleeding). If necessary, patients can also undergo a platelet transfusion to increase the platelet count. Although there is a drug called thrombopoetin that may help prevent thrombocytopenia, it has so many side effects that it is rarely used for lung cancer patients. Fortunately, the chemotherapy commonly given for lung cancer rarely causes significant thrombocytopenia.

Thrombocytopenia
Low counts of platelets that may result in bruising and/or bleeding.

The effect of chemotherapy on blood counts varies widely among patients depending on the chemotherapy regimen and on the patient's individual response. For example, cisplatin and premetrexed (Alimta) rarely causes any significant drop in the counts, while gemcitabine and carboplatin cause thrombocytopenia, and Taxol, Taxotere, and Navelbine cause neutropenia. The "targeted" agents, such as Avastin, Tarceva, and Erbitux, are targeted at pathways found only in cancer, so they rarely cause significant myelosuppression. Some patients experience only mild drops in blood counts and have few related symptoms.

If you are aware of the possible effects (and associated symptoms) of chemotherapy on your blood, you will be able to identify potential problems, alert your doctor in a timely manner, and receive more effective treatment.

72. Why am I always exhausted? What can I do for fatigue? Will the fatigue go away after my treatment is over?

There are a number of possible reasons for fatigue, particularly while on chemotherapy. One that has become popularized due to all the commercials and magazine ads recently is fatigue due to anemia from the chemotherapy. A blood test ordered by your doctor should indicate if your red blood cell (RBC) count is low enough to be the cause of your fatigue. If you are anemic, your doctor may order a blood transfusion or a medication called erythropoietin (Procrit, Epo, Aranesp). However, these medications have become much more regulated recently due to their tendency to cause blood clots. In some types of cancer, there is also data to suggest that they may shorten a cancer patient's life. For these reasons, doctors are currently able to prescribe these medications only under strict conditions. However, he or she may order a blood transfusion instead.

Another possible reason for fatigue is depression. Depression can manifest in many ways, not just an overwhelming feeling of sadness. Patients can feel despair, discouragement, lack of interest in activities they once enjoyed, change in sleeping patterns or eating patterns, and fatigue. Although anyone with cancer may experience some of these feelings some of the time, a person is clinically depressed when the depression is of such a magnitude that he or she is not able to enjoy any activities that normally bring pleasure. If you feel this might be a possibility, talk with your doctor. (See Question 81 for additional discussion of depression.)

In many cases, however, it is not easy to identify and correct the cause of fatigue. Chemotherapy and radiation are tiring—be prepared for it. Manage it by getting the rest you need and by being proactive about reducing your activities. Consider cutting back at work to part time, if at all possible. Find out in advance what your company's policy is regarding medical leaves of absence. Pamper yourself—accept help from friends. Don't worry about a messy house. Explain to your family that your body is undergoing a change and that you will not be able to do as much for the next several months. If your family has a hard time accepting this, have them come to an appointment and discuss this with your doctor or social worker.

73. I have heard stories from patients who underwent chemotherapy years ago and had terrible nausea and vomiting. Will I have a similar experience?

Almost certainly you will not. The good news is that a new class of antiemetic drugs that is much more effective in preventing nausea and vomiting has been developed over the past decade. This class of antiemetics, called HT3 blockers, can be given orally or intravenously. These drugs have had a major impact on the ability of doctors to administer—and patients to tolerate—chemotherapy. A number of these are available (Granisetron, Kytril, Anzamet, Emend, to name a few). Even the "worst" chemotherapy drugs these days often result in only some queasiness and loss of appetite for a day or two. Vomiting is much less common than it has been in the past. The bad news is that these drugs may be very expensive, particularly if taken orally, because some insurance companies do not pay for oral medications. Most oncologists will give these medications intravenously with chemotherapy, making chemotherapy considerably more tolerable than it was in the past. However, everyone is different. If you are unusually sensitive to the nausea side effects of chemotherapy and have problems with repeated vomiting episodes, call your doctor or nurse. Do not wait for your next visit! It is important not to become dehydrated—this will only make you feel worse, which will result in less fluid intake, and start a downhill spiral. If you call while you are having the problem, your doctor or nurse will alter your medications, and may even have you come to the office to receive fluids and antiemetics intravenously, which can help significantly.

Another drug which is very good at controlling nausea is the steroid dexamethasone or Decadron. Dexamethasone is much cheaper than the HT3 blockers, and is often given in combination with them. Side effects include elevation of the blood glucose for several days, so people with diabetes should take it with caution.

74. Will I lose my hair during chemotherapy or radiation? What can I do to make the experience more tolerable?

Hair loss, also known as alopecia, is one of the most common and dreaded of all cancer treatment side effects. Hair loss is difficult because it takes away your normal appearance and provides a constant reminder that you have cancer. You may feel that you are not yourself without your hair, and you may be uncomfortable or self-conscious around other people, even your family. It helps to remember that in the vast majority of cases, treatment-related hair loss is temporary, and there are things you can do to minimize the emotional and physical impact of losing your hair.

Some chemotherapy drugs are more likely to cause hair loss than others (see Table 3). Whether or not a drug causes hair loss is not an indication of how effective it is against killing cancer cells. Often, when faced with a new diagnosis of lung cancer, patients are so anxious to start treatment they forget to discuss some of the side effects with their doctor. If hair loss is important to you, tell your doctor! He or she can usually devise treatment plans which are less likely to cause hair loss without compromising how well the treatment works against the cancer.

Hair loss occurs because, in addition to cancer cells, both chemotherapy and radiation treatment adversely affect hair follicles and other fast-growing normal cells. With chemotherapy, your hair loss can range from a noticeable thinning, to patchy loss, to complete hair loss—or your hair may not be affected at all. The degree and nature of your hair loss will depend primarily on the type and amount of chemotherapy you are receiving. Your oncologist will be able to tell you what to expect, although to some extent the amount of hair loss varies from person to person. If you do lose your hair, it will begin to grow back about a month after your last treatment and take several more months to grow back fully. You shouldn't be surprised if the hair that grows back is a different texture or color than your normal hair. A change in texture is common, although over time your hair will most likely return to its original state. Extended chemotherapy treatments may also result in the loss of your body hair.

This phenomenon presents additional challenges—for example, your nose will run frequently and sweat will drip in your eyes. For some people, the loss of eyebrows and eyelashes is more disturbing than the loss of hair, which is more easily camouflaged.

With radiation, you will experience hair loss only in the area that is irradiated. Patients who receive **cranial irradiation** (radiation to the brain) almost always have total alopecia. Your hair will usually grow back, although it may be thinner than it was previously. Your hair loss may be permanent if you receive high doses of radiation.

There are several things you can do to make your experience with treatment-related hair loss more tolerable. The first thing is to prepare ahead of time. You may want to cut your hair to a short style to make the transition less traumatic. If your hair loss begins with a gradual thinning, you can reduce the rate of loss by avoiding the use of heat (curling irons, hair dryers, hot rollers) or chemicals (bleach, dyes, perms, harsh shampoos), and by using a soft brush. If your hair begins to fall out in clumps, you may find it easier and less upsetting to just shave your head at that point.

If you are planning on wearing a wig, try to get one before you start chemotherapy so you will have it when you need it. Your oncology nurse or social worker may be able to help you locate a wig shop that caters to the needs of cancer patients. Be sure to ask about the different types of wigs available and the advantages and disadvantages of each. It is possible to take your wig to your hairdresser and have it styled to look like your natural hair so that when you do make the transition, it will be less noticeable. Wigs vary greatly in cost depending on the quality of the wig you select, but your oncologist can give you a

SIDE EFFECTS OF CHEMOTHERAPY

Cranial irradiation

The exposure of the head to roentgen rays or other forms of radioactivity for therapeutic or preventive purposes.

prescription for a "hair prosthesis" that will cover some or all of the expense if you have insurance coverage. A wig is considered a deductible medical expense. If you cannot afford a wig, the American Cancer Society, CancerCare, and other cancer organizations provide wigs free of charge to those in need.

There is a wealth of choices for head coverings, including hats, scarves, and turbans. The American Cancer Society's Tender Loving Care catalog (800-850-9445 or *www.tlccatalog.org*) is a wonderful resource for these items and others designed specifically to hide hair loss. Keep in mind that there are no rules for what you should wear on your head, if anything and you should do whatever is most comfortable for you.

Understanding that your hair loss is temporary will help you to get through this tough time.

Another excellent resource for learning to cope with hair loss is the "Look Good...Feel Better" program (*www.lookgoodfeelbetter.org*) that is sponsored by the American Cancer Society and certain other nonprofit organizations. The program offers workshops in skin care, makeup, hair and nail care, and the use of wigs and headwear. They provide many useful tips for coping with head and body hair loss and provide free samples to take home. If you are not comfortable attending the program yourself, a friend or relative can go for you, or you can ask to see the program video.

Understanding that your hair loss is temporary will help you to get through this tough time.

75. I have numbness and pain in my fingers and toes that my doctor calls peripheral neuropathy. Is there an effective treatment for this condition?

Peripheral neuropathy occurs when peripheral nerves (the nerves located outside of the brain and spinal chord) are damaged. This condition can be caused by your tumor, but in most lung cancer patients it is usually caused by certain chemotherapy drugs, such as paclitaxel (Taxol) or cisplatin. Symptoms of peripheral neuropathy may include feelings of "pins and needles," numbness, and burning in the hands, feet, and legs. Motor problems, such as dropping things or problems walking, can also result from peripheral neuropathy. Sometimes a drug called Neurontin (gabepentin) can help, but this drug also has its side effects, such as fatigue. Some patients report that exercise helps with peripheral neuropathy and improves quality of life. In general, although the neuropathy rarely goes away completely, it can slowly improve with time. See Appendix A for resources to consult if you experience peripheral neuropathy.

76. What can I do about the rash I got with drugs like Tarceva or Erbitux?

Rash is one of the most common side effects for patients taking drugs like Tarceva or Erbitux (the drugs which inhibit the EGFR pathway; see Question 44) and can range from mild to severe. Typically, the rash which often looks like acne develops about 8 to 10 days after the start of treatment and affects areas above the waist. The rash is believed to be due to an inflammatory response as a result of EGFR inhibition in skin tissue and can be controlled with mild antibiotics. In most cases, the rash will improve with treatment. Tarceva rash is typically mild to moderate and can be managed by treating the rash and symptoms with a hydrocortisone cream or clindamycin gel. In some cases doxycycline or minocycline may also be prescribed.

Cases of severe rash can be unpleasant enough for some people to consider discontinuing treatment; however, recent data suggests that moderate to severe rash may be related to a better clinical outcome. You and your doctor should discuss the pros and cons and together, determine when and if it becomes severe enough to reduce the dose or interrupt the treatment.

77. Will treatment for lung cancer make me infertile? Will it affect my sex life?

Chemotherapy can cause temporary or permanent infertility. If you think you may want to have children in the future, it is extremely important that you discuss this issue with your doctor prior to treatment.

Chemotherapy can cause temporary or permanent infertility. If you think you may want to have children in the future, it is extremely important that you discuss this issue with your doctor prior to treatment. Factors that may affect fertility include the type of drug(s), the amount of drug you receive, the duration, and your individual response. Your doctor can advise you on your likelihood of infertility and on any steps that you might take to preserve your ability to have children—such as freezing your eggs or sperm for future use. Your doctor can also tell you whether you have any treatment alternatives that will not threaten your ability to have children. Radiation and surgery for lung cancer usually do not affect fertility, although to the extent that they reduce lung function, they may affect a woman's ability to carry a child. Some of the treatment agents currently in clinical trials for lung cancer do not affect fertility; however, the fertility effects of some experimental agents may be unknown. There may be nothing you can do to preserve your ability to have children in the face of lung cancer. If you share your concerns about this vital issue with your doctor, then he or she will be better able to advise you on your choices and help you to make these difficult decisions.

Your lung cancer impacts all aspects of your life, including your sexuality. A lung cancer diagnosis may affect how you feel about yourself sexually and how your partner feels about you. The pain, fatigue, shortness of breath, and other effects of cancer and its treatment affect you physically and emotionally and most likely will have a negative impact on your sex life. Communication is your best ally for combating this undesirable side effect. Communicate with your partner to let him or her know how you are feeling and how your disease and its treatment are affecting you sexually. Ask questions of your partner to be sure that he or she is expressing his or her feelings about changes that may be occurring as a result of your cancer. Discuss what you can do to accommodate these changes, such as making mental adjustments or devising alternatives to compensate for physical limitations. Talk to your doctor to learn whether there are things you can do to improve the symptoms that are interfering with your usual sex life. If your sexual relationship with your partner becomes a source of stress or concern, do not hesitate to discuss this with your doctor. Emotions and fear about cancer can cause you or your partner to make wrong assumptions or act in ways that result in hurt feelings. They can contribute to poor communication or worsen problems that existed prior to your lung cancer diagnosis. If you and your partner are having difficulties dealing with how your cancer is affecting your sex life, do not hesitate to seek professional counseling.

78. What can I do if I have lost my appetite?

Loss of appetite is a problem for many cancer patients, and often a major source of concern for family members. Some things to consider:

- Eat small meals more frequently (rather than three meals per day).
- Although it is always best to eat a well-balanced meal, for cancer patients who are struggling with loss of appetite, consuming calories is probably more important. Concentrate on eating high-calorie and high-protein foods. A variety of nutritional supplements are available; many patients feel that they taste better cold, and may mix them with ice cream or pudding.
- Talk to a nutritionist.
- There is a medication called Megace (megesterol) that can help stimulate the appetite. Ask your doctor about it.

79. Are there long-term, permanent side effects from treatment?

Your cancer treatments cause side effects. Many of these effects are temporary and disappear shortly after your treatment ends. Others may persist for years before resolving, and some may never go away completely. There are also late effects associated with treatment—effects that can appear up to years following cessation of treatment. It helps to be aware of these long-term and late effects so that you can incorporate this information into your treatment decisions. It is also important that you bring up these issues with your doctor so that, if at all possible, steps can be taken to eliminate or improve these treatment-related problems. As cancer patients are surviving longer, more is becoming known about these long-term health issues. This increased awareness helps patients to recognize these effects, and seek treatment and/or proper follow-up care. Advances in cancer care are also bringing about more effective treatments with fewer adverse effects.

The following list describes some of the long-term and late effects associated with standard lung cancer treatments. Keep in mind that some patients do not experience any long-term problems as a result of their treatment, although it is more common that you will have some lingering effects. If you experience chronic long-term pain as a result of your cancer treatment, you should not "learn to live with it"—ask your doctor for a referral to a pain clinic.

- *Surgery.* Depending on the extent of your surgery, you will likely have reduced lung function, creating physical limitations. This function may improve over time as your remaining lung tissue expands, but it may never return to presurgery capacity. You may also have numbness and nerve pain at and around the surgical site. Other reported late effects include muscle and bone pain and heartburn/reflux, resulting from shifts in your musculo-skeletal system and esophagus following lung surgery.
- *Chemotherapy.* Peripheral neuropathy is a common long-term effect of cisplatin or Taxol chemotherapy (see Question 75). Hearing loss or ringing in the ears is experienced occasionally with high doses of cisplatin. Permanent damage to fertility is possible. Some patients also report a reduction in mental function ("fuzzy thinking" and problems with memory) that is frequently referred to as "chemo brain." It

is not uncommon for patients to experience fatigue that persists long after chemotherapy has ended. Some drugs can cause permanent kidney (cisplatin), and heart (Doxorubicin) damage as well as increase the risk of a second malignancy, such as leukemia. Fortunately, these are extremely rare.

- *Radiation Therapy.* Radiation to the chest can cause permanent scarring in the lungs (**radiation fibrosis**), thereby creating significant long-term breathing problems for some patients. In rare cases, patients can also experience damage to the heart or spine, or scarring of the esophagus, causing problems swallowing. These serious effects are becoming even less common as advances in technology enable far greater precision in delivering radiation to lung tumors while sparing healthy tissue.

Radiation fibrosis

Scarring of the lungs from radiation.

PART EIGHT

Coping with Symptoms of Lung Cancer

Can my shortness of breath be controlled?

What can I do to relieve pain?

Am I at risk for a blood clot?
What is a pulmonary embolism?

More . . .

80. Can my shortness of breath be controlled?

There are many causes of shortness of breath, and how to manage it will depend upon the cause. For example, if the shortness of breath is due to a pleural or pericardial effusion, the fluid can be removed to restore breathing capacity (see Question 84). Shortness of breath caused by emphysema or COPD can be managed with inhalers and antibiotics, and pneumonia with antibiotics.

There are several ways to relieve shortness of breath if it is due to the tumor blocking an airway. Radiation is often used to reduce the tumor, thereby relieving the obstruction or blockage. If the patient has already had maximal radiation, a **stent** can sometimes be placed. A stent is a device that looks similar to a hollow tube, which is inserted via bronchoscopy into the airway that is being blocked or crushed by the tumor. Other ways of relieving the obstruction include **brachytherapy**. Brachytherapy is a method of delivering a "seed" of a radioactive agent into the tumor that is blocking the airway.

Sometimes shortness of breath cannot be controlled using these methods. In these cases, the patient's shortness of breath symptoms can be managed with:

- *Oxygen.* Portable oxygen carriers that allow patients to be mobile are available.
- *Medications, particularly morphine.* Morphine reduces the uncomfortable sensation of breathlessness, so although a person's body is not getting enough oxygen, the brain does not interpret it this way. Morphine can be given in a number of ways (see Question 82).
- *An anti-anxiety medication,* such as lorazepam (Ativan), will also help to relieve your feelings of breathlessness.

Stent

A hollow tube that can be inserted via bronchoscopy into the airway to prevent it from being blocked or crushed by the tumor.

Brachytherapy

Internal radiation therapy that involves placing "seeds" of radioactive material near or in the tumor.

81. Could I be depressed?

Depression is a common condition in lung cancer patients. Although patients who have a history of depression are most susceptible, many people who have never before experienced psychiatric problems may develop depression following a lung cancer diagnosis. Even though it is normal and natural to feel sad and down about the diagnosis, sometimes the feelings of sadness become so overwhelming that they take on a life of their own and become a problem in and of themselves. Patients can become so discouraged, hopeless, or full of despair that they are unable to enjoy their family or the little things in life. If you find yourself sitting at home all the time, no longer interested in your usual activities or in getting out of the house, withdrawing from your family, spending all your time in bed, and so on, you may be depressed. The good news is that most depression is treatable—and with medications that are usually well tolerated with minimal side effects. The bad news is that it frequently goes undiagnosed.

Depression is a common condition in lung cancer patients.

Several factors complicate the process of diagnosing depression in cancer patients. For example, many of the symptoms of depression (such as changes in eating and sleeping habits) are also symptoms associated with cancer and its treatment. Also, patients often do not openly share emotional symptoms—a major component of the depression diagnosis—with their doctors. If you think you might be depressed, it is very important that you discuss this possibility with your doctor. If your doctor does diagnose depression, he or she can treat you or refer you to a psychiatrist for further evaluation and treatment. Most frequently, cancer patients have reactive depression. Reactive depression is of limited duration and can be helped with counseling. Major depression is more severe and long lasting, and treatment most often includes medication, such as antidepressants. When depression is treated effectively, patients experience relief from distressing symptoms and are better able to cope with their cancer and the demands of cancer treatment. Recognizing the signs of depression early will help to quickly diagnose and successfully treat it.

Sometimes patients are unwilling to undergo treatment for depression, thinking that it represents a sign of weakness, and that they should be able to control their feelings. Nothing could be further from the truth. When you are hungry, you cannot trick your mind into thinking you are not. When you have to go to the bathroom, you cannot trick your mind into thinking you do not. If you are depressed, why would you be able to trick your mind into thinking that you are not?

82. What can I do to relieve my pain?

First and most importantly, talk to your doctor. He or she cannot know you are in pain unless you speak up. Advocate for yourself: if one medication is not effective in relieving your pain, or is having a lot of side effects, tell your doctor. Do not wait until your next appointment—give the office a call. If they do not call back within a reasonable period of time, call again. You deserve to have relief from pain, and your doctor and nurse would agree with you if you let them know.

Everyone feels pain differently. Your doctor and nurse will often ask you to rate the pain on a scale of 1 to 10, with 0 being no pain and 10 being very severe pain. Some patients agonize over this question, struggling with the difference between a four or a five, and they should not. There is no wrong or right answer, and your nurse or doctor will not quiz you regarding fine differences. This pain scale is simply a general way to determine whether your pain is getting better or worse.

There are many medications for pain. Typically, physicians manage mild pain with non-opioid medications, such as acetaminophen (Tylenol), or nonsteroidal anti-inflammatory drugs (NSAIDs), such as Motrin or Advil. Some type of opioid is usually required for moderate pain. Commonly used preparations include combinations of acetaminophen or NSAIDs with oxycodone or hydrocodone (e.g., Percoset, Vicodan, and Lortab), administered every six hours. Severe pain may require morphine or hydromorphine. Sometimes patients with severe pain may need to be hospitalized for intravenous morphine to quickly control the pain and to determine how much oral morphine they will need as an outpatient.

There are two major types of pain pills—short acting and long acting. Short acting pills typically last about 6 hours, and are generally used for pain that is mild, occurs occasionally, or comes and goes. Long acting pain pills build up to a low but steady level in the blood. They may take a day or two to build up to an effective level, so don't expect them to work right away. Short-acting pills are used to treat the pain you have at the time; long-acting pain pills are used to prevent it from occurring (or if it does occur, reduce its intensity).

Short-acting pain pills are taken on an "as-needed" basis. Since long-acting pain pills take awhile to build up in the bloodstream, they must be taken on a very regular basis, whether you are having pain or not.

Many patients feel they shouldn't have to take pain pills. Not so! You will do much better in the long run if you conserve your strength to fight the cancer instead of the pain. Remember—you don't get "brownie points" for putting up with pain.

Unfortunately, misconceptions about pain medications can sometimes prevent patients from taking these drugs or even talking to their doctor about pain relief. Some common misconceptions include:

- I'm afraid of getting addicted to morphine.

  Don't be. Numerous studies have shown that cancer patients in pain do not get mentally addicted to these drugs. They do not exhibit drug-seeking behavior and are able to be weaned off the medications without difficulty once the cause of the pain is controlled.

- I want to save morphine for when the time comes when I really need it.

  Don't. Numerous studies have also shown that patients do not become "tolerant" to these drugs—that is, they do not find themselves requiring more and more pain medications for the same level of pain.

- OK, but I'll still try to get away with taking as few pills as possible.

  Don't. These pain medications are much, much better at preventing pain than taking it away once it starts. These pain medications are designed to be taken on a regular basis, whether you are having pain at that time or not.

- Won't morphine make me woozy and lightheaded?

  It might, but these are side effects that usually go away with repeated treatments. If you have this problem, try starting at a lower dose and slowly working your way up to allow your body to get used to it. If this doesn't work, tell your doctor, and he or she will try a different preparation. Although it varies a lot, some people have more of one kind of side effect on one type of pill than they do with another.

- I'm afraid to take morphine because codeine makes me so constipated.

  This is one of the major problems with these drugs. It is extremely important to try to prevent the constipation—it is much harder to correct constipation after it has already occurred. Talk to your nurse or doctor about the various types of medications recommended to prevent constipation. Typically, most patients start by taking a laxative or stool softener at the same time that they take their pain medications. If you become constipated, try adding milk of magnesia. If that does not work, ask your doctor about taking the same type of medications that are used in preparation for a colonoscopy, such as sorbitol, "Go-Lytly," or magnesium citrate.

When using these medications, it is important to know that this is an area where the "art" of medicine comes in. Everyone is different, so "play around" with the timing, amount, and combinations of these medications until you have a combination that works for you.

- *What are other side effects of codeine and morphine?*

  Another possible side effect is nausea. Like constipation, if it cannot be managed with medications, ask your doctor to switch you to another type of preparation. Itching is a relatively rare side effect that can also usually be managed with medication.

- *What is the difference between codeine and morphine?*

  Codeine, morphine, oxycodone, hydrocodone, etc., all fit into a class of very similar drugs called opioids. The codeine derivatives—codeine, oxycodone, hydrocodone—tend to be less potent than morphine or its derivatives (hydromorphine, Dilaudid), which simply means that you have to take more of them to get the same effect. They all have the same side effects, though.

- *What is the maximum dose of morphine someone can take?*

  The short answer is, "there is no one maximal dose—it depends on the individual." The side effect that eventually limits the amount of these medications one can take is **respiratory depression**—slowing of breathing. However, most people are able to tolerate very high doses of opioids as long as the dose is increased gradually. A dose that would have very severe side effects in a person who has never taken these drugs may not faze a person who has been on them a while. So, even though patients do not become "immune" to the pain-killing properties of these medications, with time, they often become tolerant of the side effects.

- *I hate taking pills, period.*

  That is understandable; however, this is a time when the benefits may be far greater than any risks or concerns you may have about a pill. If you have difficulty swallowing pills, you can ask your doctor about a "fentanyl patch." This is a small piece of a plastic-like tape that contains a medication called fentanyl (or Duragesic). This medication gets absorbed through the skin over a 72-hour period of time, so the patch needs to be changed about once every three days.

- *What is the difference between oxycodone and OxyContin?*

  Oxycodone is a derivative of codeine—its effects usually last about six hours. OxyContin is a brand name for a long-acting preparation of oxycodone. There are a number of long-acting pain preparations, including OxyContin, MS Contin, Oromorph, among others. All of these medications are coated with a special substance that allows the medication to be slowly absorbed over many hours. The advantage of these medications is that they can greatly reduce the number and frequency of short-acting pain pills one has to take.

Respiratory depression

Slowing of breathing.

For these medications to work well, they have to be taken on a regular schedule. Because they get slowly absorbed, it may take several days for them to start to work. In the meantime, you can continue to take your "short-acting" pain pills. Indeed, many people have to take a short-acting pain pill occasionally for "breakthrough" pain.

Because they take longer to work, you may not feel any effects from these medications for a day or two. Therefore, it is important to take these medications whether you are having pain or not. Like their short-acting counterparts, the long-acting preparations are better at preventing pain than at relieving it, and because they take so long to work, you do not want to suffer tomorrow for not having taken one today. One way of looking at this is that the pill you take today will not be felt until tomorrow.

- *I'm afraid to take these medications, especially OxyContin, after all the stuff I've read about in the newspapers.*

Don't be. Opioids, when taken for the appropriate reasons by careful individuals, are not harmful or addicting and are true "miracle drugs" for relieving pain. They only become problematic or addicting when used inappropriately by people who are not in pain.

OxyContin in particular has been in the press lately. OxyContin is oxycodone (the same medication found in Percoset or Roxicet), but it is somewhat more concentrated. It comes in a preparation that allows the drug to be released slowly over 8 to 12 hours. Some addicts are breaking the pills open and then taking the amount of opioid that is intended to be used over 12 hours all at once. When used appropriately, OxyContin can be very helpful for lung cancer patients.

- *I've tried all these medications, they don't seem to work and I have too many side effects. I'm afraid nothing more can be done.*

Not so. Many times pain medication can be much more effectively controlled if it is given continuously through an IV pump. This small device, about the size of a cassette tape recorder, can be easily carried around with you, allowing you to live at home and perform your usual activities.

If your doctor is not able to effectively manage your pain, ask for a referral to a pain specialist or a palliative care doctor. They are experts in dealing with the various medications. In addition, they may know whether an injection or nerve block may be helpful.

If your doctor is not able to effectively manage your pain, ask for a referral to a pain specialist or a palliative care doctor.

83. Am I at risk for a blood clot? What is a pulmonary embolism?

A blood clot that occurs in a deep-lying vein in the leg or pelvis is known as a **deep vein thrombosis (DVT)**. If the blood clot breaks off and travels up through the heart and into the lungs, it is called a **pulmonary embolism (PE)**. A pulmonary embolism is a potentially serious condition, because if it is a large blood clot, it can block off a blood vessel going to the lung and cause significant problems with breathing, or even death.

Deep vein thrombosis (DVT)

A blood clot occurring in a deep-lying vein in the leg or pelvis.

Pulmonary embolism (PE)

A blood clot that travels to the lungs causing full or partial blockage of one or both pulmonary arteries.

Lots of things can cause DVT, particularly in the elderly, including poor circulation, sitting for long periods of time, or being bedridden following surgery. Cancer patients have a higher tendency to get blood clots, probably because some tumors make substances which make the blood more susceptible to clotting. (Clotting is a "paraneoplastic syndrome"—see Question 8)

To prevent DVT from happening, your doctor may put you on an anticoagulant (anti-clotting drug), such as coumadin (Warfarin) or heparin. Contrary to popular opinion, these drugs do not cause the blood clot to dissolve. Instead, they prevent the blood clot from becoming even bigger, allowing it to shrivel up and become "glued" to the wall of the vessel. Although coumadin can work well in some cancer patients, in others it does not. Those patients often need to be treated with heparin. Heparin can be administered in several ways. Until recently, patients were often admitted for intravenous heparin. More recently, low-molecular-weight heparin (such as Lovanox) has become available, which can be administered once or twice per day as an injection just under the skin. Please note that the commonly used phrase, "thinning the blood" is not quite accurate. These medications do not make the blood thinner. They make the blood less likely to clot, allowing the body to take care of the clot as previously described.

Please note that the commonly used phrase, "thinning the blood" is not quite accurate.

84. What are pleural or pericardial effusions and how are they managed?

A pleural effusion is a collection of fluid between the outside of the lung and the chest wall (the **pleural space**). The lung is covered with a thin membrane called the **visceral pleura**, and the inside of the chest wall is covered with a thin membrane called the **parietal pleura**. Normally, the outside of the lung is touching the chest wall, and the space between the visceral and parietal pleura is virtually non-existent. However, if there are tumor cells on either the visceral pleura, or the parietal pleura, they can become "irritated" and cause fluid formation.

Other conditions besides cancer can cause fluid accumulation in the pleural space, including congestive heart

Pleura

A membrane surrounding the lung (**visceral pleura**) and lining the chest wall (**parietal pleura**).

Pleural space

The area between the outside of the lung and the inside of the chest wall.

Visceral pleura

A membrane surrounding the lung.

Parietal pleura

A membrane lining the chest wall.

failure or pneumonia. To prove that the pleural effusion is indeed due to cancer, your doctor will sample some of the fluid so it can be examined under a microscope by the pathologist. This is typically done as an out-patient procedure by numbing the skin with a topical anesthetic, and then inserting a small needle into the chest and draining out some of the fluid.

One of the reasons pleural effusion is significant for lung cancer patients (in addition to the breathing problem it can cause) is that it exists in a "free-flowing" space. For example, when you stand up, the fluid settles to the bottom of the lung. When you lie on your side, it flows to the side and "layers out" along the side. If you were to stand on your head, it would flow to the top of the lung. As it flows, it can spread any cancer cells that might be floating within it, thus "seeding" other areas of either the visceral or parietal pleura. Because the fluid spreads the cancer cells around so extensively, local therapy, such as surgery and radiation, is usually not possible.

In most people, accumulation of some fluid in this area is not a problem. Some people, however, can experience shortness of breath, particularly if the pleural effusion is quite large. When it gets large, patients may also experience an uncomfortable sensation of fullness or discomfort in the chest, as well as a cough.

Thoracentesis

A procedure that uses a needle to remove fluid from the space between the lung and the chest wall.

The pleural effusion can be removed in an outpatient procedure called a **thoracentesis** (**Figure 3**). In this procedure, a needle is inserted in the back between two ribs. It is attached to a tube that drains the fluid into a bottle or bag. The procedure is relatively painless. The skin is numbed with lidocaine before the needle is inserted, so you will feel the needle to numb the area. After that, most patients do not feel anything, with the possible exception of a cough or vague discomfort if a lot of fluid is removed. These effects are due to the lung re-expanding.

If the fluid keeps reaccumulating, your doctor may recommend a procedure called **pleurodesis**. Although there are several ways of doing this, they are all based upon the principle of draining the lung very, very dry, and then inserting some medication into the space where the fluid once was between the chest wall and lung. This medication is supposed to irritate the covering of the lung and the inside of the chest wall, which in turn is supposed to cause scar tissue (or fibrosis) to form between the two, thus serving as a type of "glue" to keep the surfaces stuck together. There are a number of different ways of doing this; the size of chest tube, the choice of medication, and whether the tube is inserted in the operating room or at the bedside will vary depending on local practices.

Pleurodesis

A procedure to prevent recurrence of pleural effusion by draining the fluid and inserting medication into the pleural space.

Regardless of exactly how the procedure is done, several points should be kept in mind. First, the procedure doesn't always work. This may be because it is impossible to get the pleural space dry enough, or because sometimes the lung will not re-expand. In addition, getting the pleural space as dry as possible often involves between 5–10 days in the hospital, usually with a chest tube inserted. For these reasons, most oncologists do not recommend pleurodesis unless it becomes clear that a patient is going to need repeated thoracentesis.

Sometimes, if a pleurodesis does not work, or if a patient chooses not to undergo the procedure, the surgeon can insert a small, semi-permanent tube called a **Pleurex catheter** into the pleural space that drains to the outside (Figure 3). Fluid can then be drained periodically as it accumulates. Once in place, the tube is painless and cannot be seen under clothing.

Pleurex catheter

Provides symptomatic relief of dyspnea related to recurrent pleural effusions.

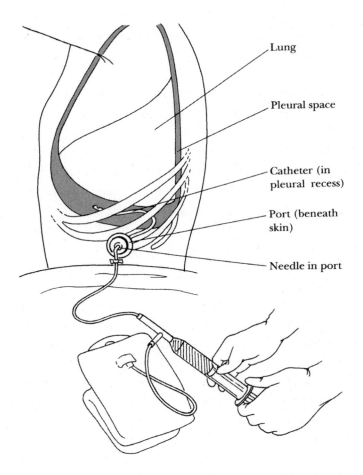

Lung

Pleural space

Catheter (in pleural recess)

Port (beneath skin)

Needle in port

Figure 3 Thoracentesis via an implanted port.

Reprinted from Yarbro CH, Frogge MH, Goodman M, Groenwald SL: *Cancer Nursing: Principles and Practice*, Sixth Ed. Copyright © 2005, Jones and Bartlett Publishers, LLC.

Pericardium

A double-layered serous membrane that surrounds the heart.

Pericardial effusion

Accumulation of fluid inside the sac (**pericardium**) that surrounds the heart.

Just as the lungs are covered with a thin membrane called the visceral pleura, the heart is covered with a thin membrane called the **pericardium**. A **pericardial effusion** is fluid that accumulates between the heart and the pericardium. Sometimes, this fluid can hinder the heart from beating effectively, and it too may need to be drained in a manner similar to the pleural fluid.

85. Is my cough something I should worry about?

Cough is a common symptom that can be due to a number of causes, including lung cancer, infection, smoking, and asthma, among others. If you have a persistent cough, you should tell your doctor. Be prepared to tell him or her how long you have had your cough, when and how often your cough occurs, whether your cough produces mucus (and if it does, what color the mucus is), and whether your cough is associated with shortness of breath, wheezing or fevers. In the majority of cases, your doctor will be able to diagnose and treat your cough effectively with therapy specific for its cause. Persistent coughs can range from a minor annoyance to a major source of fatigue and discomfort for lung cancer patients. Because effective treatment is available for most coughs, and because cough may be a symptom of a serious condition, it makes sense to seek medical attention for persistent cough. If at any time you cough up blood or see blood in your sputum (i.e., the mucus and other material that you cough up from your lungs), you should call your doctor's office immediately.

If at any time you cough up blood or see blood in your sputum (i.e., the mucus and other material that you cough up from your lungs), you should call your doctor's office immediately.

PART NINE

Living with Lung Cancer

How should I change my diet following a lung cancer diagnosis? Should I take dietary supplements? Can diet affect my survival from lung cancer?

If I smoke, is there any reason to quit? How can I quit smoking while dealing with the stress of lung cancer?

Should I be exercising?

More . . .

86. How should I change my diet following a lung cancer diagnosis? Should I take dietary supplements? Can diet affect my survival from lung cancer?

Many patients wonder whether changing their diet will improve their outcome. Frequently, patients will hear from friends and family that certain diets or foods will make a critical difference in their survival: "drink tons of green tea, it will cure your disease," or "stay away from sugar, it will feed your tumor." Although some studies have shown that people who consume diets high in fruits and vegetables have a lower risk of developing lung cancer, there is no conclusive evidence that changing your diet after you have been diagnosed with cancer can affect long-term survival.

Although some studies have shown that people who consume diets high in fruits and vegetables have a lower risk of developing lung cancer, there is no conclusive evidence that changing your diet after you have been diagnosed with cancer can affect long-term survival.

This does not mean there is no reason to pay attention to your diet. Eating a healthy diet is good for you and can certainly be beneficial when you are fighting a life-threatening disease. Eating affects how you feel, your energy level, and your overall health. The American Cancer Society's nutrition recommendations include: 1) Eat five or more servings of fruits and vegetables each day; 2) choose whole grains over processed (refined) grains and sugars; 3) limit consumption of red meats, particularly those that are high in fat and are processed; and 4) limit consumption of alcoholic beverages, if you drink at all. Of course, if you are suffering from cancer or treatment-induced weight loss, then you have special dietary needs and your doctor will advise you on what you can do to gain weight, or you can ask your doctor to refer you to a dietician or nutritionist.

There is also no definitive evidence that dietary supplementation can affect your lung cancer. If you do choose to take supplements, alert your doctor so that he or she can advise you as to whether the supplements might interfere with your cancer treatments. It is a good idea to take a multivitamin to ensure you are getting your minimum daily requirements of vitamins and minerals necessary for good health.

87. If I smoke, is there any reason to quit? How can I quit smoking while dealing with the stress of lung cancer?

Yes, there are strong and compelling reasons for smokers to quit following a lung cancer diagnosis. The National Cancer Institute has found that cancer patients who continue to smoke may reduce the effectiveness of their treatment and increase the likelihood of a second cancer. There is also reason to believe that continued smoking may worsen the side effects of treatment, put you at increased risk for complications following lung surgery, and decrease your survival time. One study conducted in small cell lung cancer patients found that survival correlated with smoking status: the patients who continued to smoke after their diagnosis had the poorest survival; the patients who quit at diagnosis fared better; and the patients who had quit on average 2.5 years prior to diagnosis survived the longest.

The National Cancer Institute has found that cancer patients who continue to smoke may reduce the effectiveness of their treatment and increase the likelihood of a second cancer.

Consider how the following health benefits of smoking cessation might affect you at this critical time in your life:

- Your circulation will improve.
- Your pulse rate and blood pressure which are abnormally high while smoking will return to normal.
- Your sense of taste and smell will return.

- Your breathing will become easier.
- Your risk of developing infections such as pneumonia (a common cause of death in people with lung cancer) is reduced.
- Your risk of developing other smoking-related disease, including heart disease and other lung disease, are reduced.

It is never too late to quit. Even following your lung cancer diagnosis, smoking cessation will have a positive impact on your health, your quality of life and, possibly, your survival.

Your challenge is to motivate yourself to quit smoking during an extremely stressful time in your life. For some people this is easy—just hearing the words "lung cancer" is sufficient motivation. For others, the quitting process becomes even more difficult because smoking relieves the anxiety that comes with having lung cancer. Although quitting smoking is hard work, (nicotine is very addicting) there are proven methods available to help you. The Surgeon General recommends **nicotine replacement therapy** (in patch, gum, inhaler, and nasal spray forms) and the antidepressant, Bupropion SR (Zyban), as treatments that increase long-term quit rates. The effectiveness of these drugs is further increased with counseling, including behavior modification therapy, problem-solving/skills training, and social support. The more intense the counseling, the more likely you are to quit.

Your doctor can help you to find the combination of cessation methods that will work best for you and advise you on smoking cessation programs that are available in your community. Remember that you may have to make several attempts before you succeed—don't get discouraged. Keep trying and don't try to go it alone—seek

Nicotine replacement therapy

Smoking cessation method that uses nicotine substitutes in various forms, including a patch, gum, inhaler, or nasal spray.

support when you need it. For information on organizations, programs, and Internet resources to help you stop smoking, (see Appendix A).

Not everyone who smokes and is diagnosed with lung cancer is able to quit smoking. Although there are definite health benefits, there are also understandable reasons why it is not possible for some patients with advanced lung cancer to quit. Scientists are learning that addiction to nicotine in some patients is due to chemical imbalances in the brain, making some patients more addicted than others. In those cases, it is important for the patient and the patient's family to let go of any guilt or anger over smoking. Conflict over smoking only serves to add additional stress on top of an already stressful existence. If you or your family cannot come to terms with your continued smoking, you should seek professional counseling to resolve this divisive issue.

If you or your family cannot come to terms with your continued smoking, you should seek professional counseling to resolve this divisive issue.

88. Should I be exercising?

Exercise can improve both your physical and mental health. It is no different when you have lung cancer. The general benefits credited to exercise—increased strength and energy, elevated mood—are even more desirable when you are battling cancer. The problem is that both your cancer and its treatment make exercise more difficult. However, studies in breast cancer patients have demonstrated that a 20- to 30-minute walking program (5 to 6 times per week) during chemotherapy or radiation therapy helps to decrease levels of fatigue and emotional distress, and increase sleep quality, physical functioning, and quality of life. In some cases, exercise can provide both relief and distraction. So there are compelling reasons to get out of your chair and walk—even if it's just a few more steps than yesterday.

A useful exercise for lung cancer patients to learn is called abdominal breathing. Abdominal breathing can help to expand your lungs and increase the flow of oxygen. This is especially desirable for patients who have had surgery to remove a portion of their lung(s). Pulmonary therapists can teach you abdominal breathing and provide additional exercises to maximize your breathing capacity. Physical therapists can show you exercises to increase your upper body strength and range of motion. These exercises are not just for rehabilitation; they can help you with the long term physical changes that result from surgery. If your surgeon has not given you a referral to a physical therapist, ask for one.

89. What should I know about stress and the immune system? How does stress affect my survival and my ability to cope with my disease? Can complementary therapies help to reduce my stress?

A lung cancer diagnosis brings a pile of additional stress into your life: the stress of knowing you have a life-threatening disease; the stress of deciding what treatment to pursue; the stress of the treatment itself; the stress brought on by the impact of your cancer on the lives of your family and on your daily routine; the stress of explaining your lung cancer to your family and friends (and of dealing with their reactions); the stress of how your lung cancer affects your ability to work and your financial situation—the list of cancer-related stressors is seemingly endless. Stress is an undesirable condition that can negatively affect both your physical and mental well-being. Stress can take away your ability to relax, seek peace of mind, and enjoy life. Although there is no evidence that stress will cause your tumor to grow faster or lessen your chances for long-term survival, it makes sense that someone who is highly stressed experiences a reduced quality of life.

The first step in reducing the stress in your life is to identify your stressors, i.e., those things causing you stress. Make a list of everything you can think of that brings on anxiety or causes you to feel additional stress, whether cancer-related or not. Take time to think about how you can eliminate these stressors from your life or reduce the negative impact they have on you. Be creative. Delegate whenever possible. Don't be shy about asking for help or backing out of commitments made prior to your diagnosis. People will understand that lung cancer has changed your priorities and that you now have to focus on your health. Don't be tied to activities that have more of a negative effect on your life than a positive effect. You'll be amazed at how much stress you can eliminate when you sit down and take stock of the nonessentials in your life.

The ultimate challenge for most patients, however, is the stress brought on by family and financial obligations, and by the physical and emotional consequences of having lung cancer. If your ability to cope with these responsibilities interferes with your daily functioning, you should seek professional counseling. Complementary therapies can also help you to manage your stress. If you can find activities that help you to relax and feel less stressed, you will be better able to cope with the challenges that come your way. Complementary therapies used by cancer patients to reduce stress include relaxation and meditation, exercise programs such as yoga and tai chi, hypnotherapy, biofeedback, massage, and art and music therapy. Many cancer centers offer these types of therapies to patients. For further information on complementary therapies, (see Question 100).

90. What about returning to work? I am worried about being able to function at 100 percent. What are my rights?

Returning to work after time off for cancer treatment can be both physically and psychologically challenging. You may have physical limitations as a result of your treatment, such as breathing problems and fatigue, which make full-time employment difficult. You may also worry about the reactions of your co-workers to your cancer and dread answering their questions about your health. The process of returning to work is different for everyone. Whether yours will be a smooth transition depends on a number of factors: the extent of your physical limitations; your comfort level in sharing information about your cancer with your coworkers; how supportive (and flexible) your employer is about your needs; your attitude toward your work; and the physical and emotional demands of your job.

Before you negotiate the terms of your return to work, it is important that you are aware of your rights and protections under both federal and state law. The Americans with Disabilities Act (ADA) prohibits discrimination by both public and private employers against qualified workers with disabilities or histories of disabilities. The Federal Rehabilitation Act of 1973 ensures that federal employers or companies receiving federal funds cannot discriminate against cancer survivors (among others) in hiring practices, promotions, transfers, and layoffs. You may have additional employment protections depending upon the laws in your state.

Planning for your return to work can make a difference: know your rights, consider how you will respond to questions from coworkers, and think ahead about what accommodations you might require on a short- or long-term basis so that you will be prepared to discuss your options with your employer. See Question 100 for resources that can assist you in determining your employment rights as a cancer survivor, provide information on how to ease your transition back to work, and direct you to resources you can turn to in the event that you suffer workplace discrimination.

91. What happens when my treatment ends? Why don't I feel happy—or at least relieved?

If your treatment has been successful, and there is no evidence of your lung cancer, you have reason to celebrate. Your hopes for long-term survival, and for a normal life with your friends and family, are closer to becoming a reality. Yet, while you may feel happy on one level, you may also feel anxious on another. This is not unusual. With lung cancer, the fear of recurrence is always there. Active treatment may have given you a sense of security; however, now that your treatment has stopped, your level of anxiety may have increased. You may feel somewhat abandoned—most likely you have become used to frequent office or hospital visits, and have developed close relationships with your doctors, nurses, and the receptionists, and now you are not going to see them for awhile. You may also be coping with treatment-related side effects—breathing issues, fatigue, peripheral neuropathy—that interfere with daily life. Your support system may disappear when your treatment ends. Family and friends may hear your good news and stop inquiring after you—the cards, e-mails, phone calls, and visits that had uplifted you in the past may become less frequent or stop entirely. This is a time of transition. It is not surprising that many lung cancer survivors find it difficult to carry on with their lives after finishing treatment.

A lung cancer support group may be helpful to you at this time. Here, you may find other lung cancer survivors who are facing similar circumstances. You will also be able to reach out to newly diagnosed patients. This effort to help others can make you feel good about yourself and remind you about how far you have come. If your anxiety causes you to feel depressed or interferes with your functioning, you should talk to your doctor and ask whether counseling or medication might help to lessen your distress. This might be a good time to see a therapist for ideas about how to cope better. You should also let your family and friends know that you still need their support even though you are no longer in treatment. They may assume everything is OK unless you take the time to explain your ongoing needs.

The most important thing you can do during this time is to be vigilant about your follow-up care. Although follow-up care for lung cancer varies among doctors, you should be aware of and comfortable with your doctor's recommendations for office visits, blood tests, and scans. If you are worried about recurrence, ask your doctor if there are any chemoprevention trials that might be appropriate for you (see Questions 59 and 60). In addition to your lung cancer-related concerns, you should discuss "well care" with your doctor. It is important that you take good care of your health (good nutrition, exercise) so that you can be strong in your survival.

The most important thing you can do during this time is to be vigilant about your follow-up care.

What will be most effective for resolving your emotional distress, and sometimes also your treatment side effects, is the passage of time. As each day passes, you will feel more comfortable with your status as a lung cancer survivor. You will adjust to the emotional, physical, and social changes brought about by your lung cancer experience and find a new equilibrium—a new normal—that will carry you through your life.

92. What about follow-up care? How often should I be seen? What is my doctor looking for?

After you have completed treatment for your lung cancer, it is important that you receive regular follow-up care. Your doctor will want to see you to check for recurrence of your lung cancer, to manage any long-term effects from your cancer and its treatment, and to monitor for a second lung cancer or other primary cancer.

The American Society of Clinical Oncologists (ASCO) recommends the following follow-up schedule for asymptomatic (not currently showing symptoms of) lung cancer patients treated with curative intent: every 3 months during the first 2 years; every 6 months during years 3 through 5; and yearly thereafter. More frequent visits are warranted for patients with Stage III disease.

At each follow-up visit, your doctor will order certain blood tests, take a medical history, and perform a physical exam. X-rays and CT scans will be ordered regularly to monitor for recurrence in the lungs. Unfortunately, there are no standard recommendations for the frequency of these imaging studies, and practices among lung specialists vary widely. Although the brain and bone are common sites of metastasis in lung cancer, scans to detect metastatic disease (such as a brain MRI or a bone scan) are usually ordered only if symptoms are present.

The purpose of follow-up care, however, is to detect recurrence or disease at an early stage when it can be treated curatively or, if that is not possible, to begin **palliative treatment** in a timely manner. You will want to ask your doctor what symptoms you should be concerned about and under what circumstances you should report them.

Palliative treatment

Treatment given not with the intent to cure but with the intent to prolong survival and reduce symptoms from the tumor.

Even though you are at high risk of recurrence during the first few years after your diagnosis, your risk declines as time goes on. You remain at increased risk, however, for a second, totally different primary lung cancer. Watching for a second lung cancer is important because **resection** of second primaries can be successful.

Resection

Surgical removal.

Although your primary concern during your follow-up visits will undoubtedly be to make sure that your lung cancer has not recurred or that a second lung cancer has not developed, you should not hesitate to bring up other health issues that impact your quality of life. It is not unusual for patients to experience depression when their treatment stops, and you should discuss this with your doctor if you feel depressed or overly anxious and think you might benefit from counseling. Patients who have undergone chemotherapy, radiation, or surgery may experience long-term side effects that should be discussed on a regular basis so they can be properly addressed. (See Question 79 for discussion of long-term and late effects.) Do not feel that your complaints are too minor to bring up during your follow-up visits. Your quality of life is important and your doctor should work with you to address these concerns.

93. Should I get a flu shot? What about the pneumonia vaccine?

Lung infections can pose a serious and potentially deadly threat to lung cancer patients. Safe and effective vaccines are available for both influenza (the flu) and pneumococcal pneumonia, two common lung infections. Note that these vaccines protect against two very specific diseases—influenza and pneumococcal pneumonia—and therefore are not a guarantee you will not contract another respiratory illness, such as the common cold.

The flu shot is administered yearly, most optimally in October or November. You can get the pneumonia vaccine at any time, and revaccination is recommended after 5 years. Don't wait to ask your doctor about getting vaccinated; it could save your life.

Don't wait to ask your doctor about getting vaccinated; it could save your life.

LIVING WITH LUNG CANCER

PART TEN

If Treatment Fails

How do I decide if it's time to stop treatment?

What is hospice?

What can I do to prepare for my death?

More . . .

94. How do I decide when it's time to stop treatment?

Deciding when to stop treatment is an extremely difficult and personal decision that no one can make for you. Each person must come to this point on his or her own terms—there is no one way for you to decide. Often decisions to stop treatment come about when the side effects of treatment outweigh any potential benefit. However, this decision is deeply personal and can result from a number of circumstances occurring at the same time. Most importantly, it should be based on your values and beliefs. You may seek counsel from the people who have helped you to make decisions along the way—this may include family members, friends, healthcare providers, spiritual advisors, and others. Family members and friends may provide guidance and support as you struggle with your decision, but you should realize that their counsel will be charged with their own emotions and views. This may create conflict and make the decision more difficult for you. They may not be "ready." On the other hand, you may find that the view of your family is in line with yours, thereby making your decision easier. Ultimately, however, it is your decision to make. There is no way to predict how you will come to a decision to stop treatment and how others will react to your decision. What matters most is that you are at peace with the decision you have made.

There is no way to predict how you will come to a decision to stop treatment and how others will react to your decision. What matters most is that you are at peace with the decision you have made.

95. What is hospice?

Hospice began as a philosophy for how end-of-life care should be provided. Today, hospice organizations provide palliative care to dying patients; usually in their homes. Hospice patients are cared for by a team that may include doctors, nurses, nursing assistants, social workers, therapists, spiritual advisors, counselors, and hospice volunteers, among others. Although most hospices do not provide 24-hour care, hospices do provide a wide range of support to the terminally ill by addressing their medical, emotional, spiritual, and practical needs as well as by providing support for family members. Typical services include providing equipment and oxygen in the home; nursing assistants to help with bathing; nursing services to administer intravenous pain medications; social worker support and grief counseling. One of the big advantages of hospice (in addition to providing equipment and medications) is that the hospice nurses act as your doctor's eyes and ears, decreasing the number of trips to the doctor for problems. In addition, they can give IV medications and fluids at home, which is much more convenient.

A primary focus of hospice care is to provide symptom relief, and hospice professionals are particularly expert at pain management. Many patients choose hospice care to ensure that their final days will be as pain-free as possible. Some hospices allow chemotherapy, providing it is given for palliative purposes; most hospices allow radiotherapy for the same reason.

Most often, hospices provide care at home, but some hospices also have in-patient hospice centers or long-term care facilities. The range and amount of hospice services available to you will depend on your local hospice and on your insurance plan. Hospice coverage is provided by Medicare, and often also by Medicaid and private insurance providers. For further information on hospice and how to locate hospice services, see the resources listed in Question 100.

Many hospices state they are for patients with less than six months to live, which of course is very scary. However, this is *not* a hard and fast rule—it is merely meant to be a "guideline." Also, you can be on Hospice and then come off if things get better.

Most hospices like to meet possible patients well in advance, even before they are needed. This allows them to meet the patient and family in a more relaxed setting, so they are not coming into an emergency situation. That way, they get to know you, your particular situation, and can describe the services they offer. Ask your doctor for a referral if you think you might need Hospice at some point.

96. What can I do to prepare for my death?

In the middle of agonizing emotions and physical challenges, patients who are dying have important decisions to make. Addressing these end-of-life issues proactively can help terminally ill patients to resolve physical, psychological, and practical challenges in a way that is consistent with personal beliefs. Hopefully this will provide some measure of comfort and peace of mind to both patient and family.

End-of-life medical care. Talk to your doctor about his or her comfort level in handling end-of-life issues. If he or she is not comfortable in handling these issues, or has done so only rarely, you might want to seek a palliative care consultation. A palliative care doctor specializes in the needs of terminally ill patients. You deserve to have symptom management and relief from pain during your final days, and you may want to consider hospice care at this time (see Question 95). It is critical that you communicate your wishes about your medical care at the end of life to your healthcare providers. **Advance directives** will allow you to prepare for the medical possibilities and assign someone who can act on your behalf, should you become unable to direct your own medical care (see Question 97). Your views on what "quality of life" and "death with dignity" mean to you are appropriate topics to discuss with both your doctors and the person you have designated to act on your behalf (also called a **healthcare proxy**).

Think about your emotional and spiritual needs. Fear or denial of approaching death, or anxiety about the dying process, is common. You may want to find someone with whom you can discuss your feelings about death and dying. This could be your doctor, your religious leader, a family member, or a close friend. Many patients also explore the meaning of their lives and of their cancer experiences during this time. This spiritual journey is important to patients, regardless of their religious background and practice.

Take care of financial affairs including making sure your will is in order. Though it is difficult to deal with these sensitive concerns, it will lessen the burdens on your family after your death.

Attend to unfinished business—settle up emotional accounts. Make amends; say your goodbyes. Spend time with those who mean the most to you.

A palliative care specialist, hospice, your doctor, or a social worker will be able to refer you to end-of-life support resources. By preparing for your eventual death, you will help yourself and your family to cope with the dying process. Many terminally ill patients worry that they will be a burden to their families. This is less likely to occur

Advance directives will allow you to prepare for the medical possibilities and assign someone who can act on your behalf, should you become unable to direct your own medical care.

IF TREATMENT FAILS

Advance directives

Legal documents that allow you to prepare for future medical possibilities and to assign someone to act on your behalf in the event you become unable to direct your own medical care.

Healthcare proxy

A person you have designated to make healthcare decisions for you in the event you become incapacitated.

when you have addressed these issues ahead of time: you'll have the peace of mind of knowing that you have done all you can to spare your family additional stress. You can then concentrate on your quality of life and on sharing time with your loved ones during your final days.

97. What are advance directives?

Advance directives are legal documents that specify your wishes regarding your future medical care. They are used in the event that you become unable to make these decisions yourself. As a patient, you have the right to accept or refuse medical treatment; advance directives protect this right.

You should familiarize yourself with these three types of advance directives:

Do Not Resuscitate (DNR) order. Your doctor may (in fact, should) ask you about a DNR order. This may be a very uncomfortable subject to discuss, but it is something everyone should think about, regardless of one's health. Your doctor wants to know whether, in the event of a cardiac or respiratory arrest (e.g., a massive heart attack or if you stop breathing, regardless of the reason), you would want "heroic" measures performed—that is, whether you would want doctors to do whatever is necessary to keep you alive. These measures could involve shocking your chest, putting in a breathing tube, or putting you on a ventilator (breathing machine) in the intensive care unit. Some considerations to keep in mind before you decide:

- How strong are you? Very weak patients rarely recover enough to eventually get off the breathing machine and leave the intensive care unit, even if it was not cancer that caused their heart or lungs to stop.

- Why did this happen? If it happened because of a complication of the lung cancer, and if the lung cancer is advanced and unlikely to be controlled, the chances of successfully coming off the ventilator are very remote.

- How difficult will it be for your family to decide when to stop trying? (Often thought of as the "When to pull the plug?" decision.)

There are several reasons why it is very important that you think about this issue and discuss it with your family before you get seriously ill:

- It is much easier to be calm and objective when talking about a "hypothetical" event.

- Very often, the heart or lungs can stop working suddenly and there is not time to have a discussion as to whether to try to revive the patient. If a DNR order has not been written, the patient will almost always be "coded," and an attempt to resuscitate the patient will be made.

This is the one type of advance directive that does not require your signature—your doctor can write an order on your chart after having discussed it with you. Also, should you decide to be "DNR," ask your doctor or nurse about a DNR bracelet. This is a small plastic band, similar to a hospital identification band, worn around the wrist that indicates you do not want to be resuscitated in the event of a cardiac or respiratory arrest. This bracelet will prevent paramedics from trying to resuscitate you should you collapse out in public.

Sometimes patients are reluctant to be made DNR, thinking that it means that no treatment will be given for anything, and that the doctor is giving up on them.

Sometimes patients are reluctant to be made DNR, thinking that it means that no treatment will be given for anything, and that the doctor is giving up on them. Nothing could be further from the truth.

Nothing could be further from the truth. DNR does NOT mean "do not treat"—the type of treatment you want for your cancer or other conditions, if any, is between you and your doctor. DNR simply means that you will not be put on a breathing machine should you have a heart attack or stop breathing.

Living will. A living will is a document in which you specify which medical treatments you do and do not want to have should you become unable to decide for yourself. Because one cannot anticipate every eventuality, most health care providers recommend a medical power of attorney rather than a living will. It is important that you discuss your living will with your doctor. Your doctor can explain any medical and ethical details that you need to know in order to make decisions about end-of-life care. The National Cancer Institute recommends that you consider the following life-sustaining measures when drawing up your living will:

- The use of life-sustaining equipment (dialysis machines, ventilators, and respirators)
- "Do not resuscitate" (DNR) orders; artificial hydration and nutrition (tube feeding)
- Withholding of food and fluids
- Palliative/comfort care
- Organ and tissue donation

A critical part of the living will process is to discuss your wishes with your family and loved ones. This will allow them to more easily understand and accept your decisions.

Durable power of attorney for health care. A durable power of attorney for health care is also known as a medical power of attorney. This type of advance directive allows you to specify a healthcare proxy—a trusted person such as your spouse or other loved one—to make medical decisions for you should you become unable to do so for yourself. You should share your general and specific views regarding life-sustaining care and end-of-life issues with the person who will be your healthcare proxy, and make sure this person will be able to make your medical decisions for you—even under circumstances in which your wishes may not be known.

Most hospitals, lawyers, and palliative care physicians recommend a durable power of attorney over a living will, because a living will can never foresee all possibilities as to what may happen to a person. If you have designated a power of attorney, however, and this person knows you well, he or she probably will know what you would want done regardless of the circumstance.

Sources for additional information on preparing advance directives can be found in the "Hospice & End-of-Life Issues" section of Appendix A. Copies of signed documents should be given to your doctor and to your healthcare proxy.

You shouldn't worry that by preparing an advance directive; you are giving up on your hope for survival or turning your lung cancer into an automatic death sentence. Ideally, everyone should have advance directives—not just people with serious or life-threatening conditions. By dealing with these difficult end-of-life issues ahead of time, and by discussing them with your family and loved ones, you will have removed a potential source of distress for them and given yourself peace of mind that your wishes will be carried out.

PART ELEVEN

Prevention, Screening, and Advocacy

Can lung cancer be prevented?
What is chemoprevention?

Is there a screening test for lung cancer?

Why has there been so little progress in fighting lung cancer? What can I do to help?

More . . .

98. Can lung cancer be prevented? What is chemoprevention?

A key to preventing lung cancer is smoking prevention and cessation. Active smoking is responsible for 85–90% of all lung cancers, and exposure to second-hand smoke accounts for a significant portion of the remaining cases. But it's incorrect to consider lung cancer as only a smoker's disease. About 15 percent of people diagnosed with lung cancer have never smoked. In addition, about half of all lung cancers in the United States occur in people who have given up smoking. Although the risk of developing lung cancer goes down with smoking cessation, it never goes away completely. A significant risk remains for 20 years or longer after quitting.

Active smoking is responsible for 85–90% of all lung cancers, and exposure to second-hand smoke accounts for a significant portion of the remaining cases.

Preventing people from smoking would no doubt result in a vast reduction in the incidence of lung cancer. Tragically, there has been little progress toward reaching this goal. Tobacco companies continue to be effective in marketing their deadly product to teenagers, who are likely to ignore the risks associated with smoking. Messages that promote smoking as a cool behavior are rampant throughout our culture, making a mockery of anti-smoking campaigns. Public health initiatives in smoking prevention have not succeeded—we need more and more effective, school-based prevention programs beginning in preschool. And children and adults who are already smoking deserve better access to resources that will help them quit. Although smoking cessation will reduce the likelihood of getting lung cancer, a smoker's risk will never be equal to that of a non-smoker. The best advice for preventing lung cancer is to never start smoking, and to avoid chronic exposure to secondhand smoke.

Other environmental hazards, such as exposure to asbestos and radon, are responsible for a small percentage of lung cancer cases. Federal safety regulations are helping to prevent exposure to these and other lung carcinogens in the workplace.

Clinical trials are underway to determine whether lung cancer can be prevented in people who are at high risk for the disease, such as current and former smokers and people with a history of lung cancer. These studies are called chemoprevention trials. They are designed to test whether natural or chemical substances can prevent cancer.

Findings from previous chemoprevention trials involving beta-carotene and alpha-tocopherol (a type of vitamin E) were discouraging. The results in some cases showed that these supplements actually increased the incidence of lung cancer in smokers. As more is learned about lung **carcinogenesis,** scientists continue to test promising chemopreventive agents. If your lung cancer is in remission, you may be a candidate for a chemoprevention trial. Ask your doctor whether this might be a good option for you. Because increased participation will help find ways to prevent lung cancer, you should encourage your family and friends who are current or former smokers to consider chemoprevention trials. For information on locating chemoprevention trials, (see Appendix A).

Carcinogenesis
The development of cancer.

99. Is there a screening test for lung cancer? Does lung cancer run in families? Is my family at increased risk for lung cancer because I have lung cancer?

It is important to first understand what a screening test is. A screening test looks at asymptomatic individuals (people without symptoms) with a particular risk factor for a disease in hopes of making an early diagnosis. Making an earlier diagnosis is not enough, however; for a screening test to be useful, the earlier diagnosis must result in fewer people dying of the disease, or at least living longer. This is different from a diagnostic test, which is done to confirm the presence of a disease in a patient who already has symptoms. Currently there is no recommended screening test for lung cancer such as exists for breast (mammography), colon (fecal occult blood and sigmoidoscopy), and prostate (prostate specific antigen [PSA]) cancers. The lack of an effective screening program for lung cancer is devastating. Without screening, lung cancer patients do not get diagnosed until they become symptomatic—when, invariably, their cancer is advanced and incurable.

Intuitively, one would think that if one could detect a cancer earlier, it would be easier to cure, and that may in fact be the case. However, lung cancer screening has been quite controversial. This is because although there are screening tests that have the potential to identify lung cancer in its early stages, there are not yet scientific studies that prove that any of these tests actually reduce **mortality** for lung cancer patients. It's important here to note the difference between mortality and survival. Survival is the amount of time a person lives after they have been diagnosed with a disease. Therefore, by definition, if you detect a disease earlier, the person's survival will appear to be longer, even if you have not instituted any treatment. Mortality, on the other hand, reflects how many patients will die of the disease.

Mortality

The number of people who die of a disease.

In the past, chest x-rays have been used for lung cancer screening on an informal basis, and there are lung cancer specialists who believe that chest x-rays done in high-risk populations find enough early cancers to justify their use as a screening test. However, most specialists feel that by the time a lung cancer has grown to the point that it can be seen on a chest x-ray, it may have already spread to other parts of the body. Randomized screening trials in the 1970s failed to show that smokers who underwent annual chest x-rays were less likely to die of lung cancer than those who did not. Therefore, the American Cancer Society, which interprets available screening data, does not recommend a chest x-ray as a screening tool for lung cancer. However, there are some scientists who now say those studies were flawed, so the debate over x-ray screening for lung cancer continues.

A promising new technology called a low-dose spiral CT scan has been shown to be better at detecting small lung abnormalities (nodules) than x-ray. However, it is not yet known whether detection of very small lung nodules will result in fewer lung cancer deaths: even though lung cancers are found when they are smaller, is it still too late? Have they already spread? Also, there is emerging data to suggest that some of the very small cancers that are found on chest CT are very slow growing, and may never harm the patient.

What is the down side to physicians routinely recommending spiral CT screening? Why not just order them on everyone? It turns out that a large percentage of people (in some studies, over 70%) have very small abnormalities on CT scans and, in most cases it is unclear what these abnormalities are. Thus, many people need to be followed with repeat CT scans for years before the radiologist feels comfortable calling abnormalities benign. The price of such screening tests may therefore be the cost to society of the intensive follow-up that most patients will have to undergo, as well as the anxiety these tests produce. In addition, there is a small risk associated with exposing people to radiation from repeat CTs if they do not need them. Furthermore, some patients end up having biopsies of what turns out to be benign lesions, and there is some risk and discomfort associated with that as well. For all these reasons, physicians are sometimes reluctant to routinely recommend screening CTs until it is proven that they prevent lung cancer deaths. A large clinical trial is underway at many medical centers throughout the world to try to better understand whether this approach is likely to reduce the individual and societal burdens of lung cancer. Currently, most insurance companies are not paying for the screening CT.

If you have friends and family who are current or former smokers, you should make them aware of screening trials for lung cancer. Other candidates for screening include individuals who have had significant exposure to environmental carcinogens, such as second-hand smoke, radon, and asbestos (in the home or in the workplace) and individuals with a family history of lung cancer. For information on locating screening trials, see Appendix A.

Does lung cancer run in families?

Some families do have a high incidence of lung cancer. Scientists are studying these families to determine why certain people are at greater risk for developing this deadly disease. It may be that in some cases, blood relatives with lung cancer share genetic mutations (abnormalities) that make them more susceptible to smoking and other environmental carcinogens. This is probably due to the fact that some people do not metabolize (neutralize and excrete) carcinogens (cancer-causing substances) in cigarette smoke as well as others, and this may be inherited. Several studies have shown that women may be more susceptible to developing lung cancer than men.

PREVENTION, SCREENING, AND ADVOCACY

Although our present understanding is limited, research into families with lung cancer is shedding light on the complex relationship among the lifestyle, environmental, and genetic factors that make up lung cancer risk.

Currently, there is no genetic test to determine risk for lung cancer. Thus, there is no way to know whether your family (particularly your siblings and children) may be at increased risk because of your lung cancer. As genetic markers for lung cancer risk continue to be identified and characterized, this may change. It makes sense for anyone with a family history of lung cancer to discuss this, and other risk factors, with his or her doctor. There are no recommendations for widespread screening for lung cancer, although a doctor may choose to do this for individuals in certain cases.

If two or more members of your family have lung cancer, you may be able to participate in a family research study. For more information, contact the Johns Hopkins National Familial Lung Cancer Registry by phone at 410-614-1910 or visit its web site at *www.path.jhu.edu/nfltr.html*.

100. Why has there been so little progress in fighting lung cancer? What can I do to help?

It is frustrating to learn that although lung cancer is the number one cancer killer of men and women, it is funded at significantly lower levels than the other common cancers. Lung cancer advocates have long argued that this disparity exists because lung cancer is associated with smoking and perceived by the public as a self-inflicted disease. This smoking stigma affects both public support and media coverage of lung cancer. It also affects the willingness of people with lung cancer to stand up and speak out about this deadly disease. Many lung cancer survivors feel guilty about their smoking and fear public scorn if they were to demand more dollars for lung cancer research. And, for many people with lung cancer, the possibility of becoming an advocate is out of the question—the sad fact is that the overwhelming majority of people with lung cancer will not survive their disease. They are too sick to advocate for themselves, and their families are too grief-stricken to spend the emotional energy. In addition, although there are numerous advocacy organizations for breast, colon, and prostate cancers, there are far fewer organizations advocating on behalf of lung cancer patients.

Nevertheless, there is reason to believe that the outlook for people with lung cancer is changing. In 2001, the National Cancer Institute (NCI) held an important meeting called the Lung Cancer Progress Review Group (PRG) Roundtable that brought together more than 100 leading scientists and clinicians along with several lung cancer advocates. The meeting resulted in a comprehensive report that put forth a national agenda for lung cancer research. In addition to identifying scientific goals and challenges, the report specifically addresses the issues of disproportionate funding and stigma ("blame the victim") as barriers to progress. You can obtain the Lung Cancer PRG report by calling 1-800-4-CANCER, or by visiting the online report: *prg.nci.nih.gov/lung/finalreport.html*.

There are countless ways that individuals can help to effect the changes necessary to make this PRG "strategy for progress" a reality. Here are a few places to start:

Familiarize yourself with lung cancer issues. Read the Lung Cancer PRG Report. Read the lung cancer information on the NCI's web site, *www.cancer.gov*. Read everything on lung cancer that you come across in the media. Think about how these issues affect you, and how they affect other lung cancer survivors, as well as people at risk for lung cancer.

Contact a lung cancer advocacy organization such as the National Lung Cancer Partnership. [See **Appendix** for contact information.] Let them know you are interested in participating in advocacy activities. Advocacy organizations initiate and coordinate efforts to influence policy and funding for lung cancer research, raise awareness of lung cancer, and increase support services for people with lung cancer.

Support lung cancer research. Breast cancer advocates have been remarkably successful in raising money for research, and many feel that this is one reason why the breast cancer cure rate has gone up. A number of lung cancer advocacy organizations raise money for research—tell your friends and family.

Let your voice be heard. Write to your representatives in Washington and to your local media about lung cancer and lung cancer issues. Volunteer to participate in school anti-smoking programs. Visit local hospitals and advocate for increased information, education and support services for lung cancer patients. Advocacy organizations can provide guidance and materials for these types of efforts and connect you with other survivors who are interested in effecting change. Remember, there is strength in numbers. Lung cancer advocates are working hard to network with each other and to follow the progress that has come about for breast, prostate, and colon cancers. Our voices are gradually becoming a chorus.

PREVENTION, SCREENING, AND ADVOCACY

Put a face on lung cancer. You do not have to become a full-time advocate to make a difference in the fight against lung cancer. Each time you identify yourself as a lung cancer survivor, you are putting a face on lung cancer. You are telling the world that people with lung cancer matter and deserve the same respect as people with other forms of cancer. You are bringing others into the lung cancer community. This is a battle we all can win together.

Appendix:
Where Can I Find
More Information?

Lung Cancer Information

American Society of Clinical Oncology (ASCO)
1900 Duke Street, Suite 200, Alexandria, VA 22314
Phone: 703-299-0150
Web site: *www.cancer.net*
ASCO is a professional organization for cancer doctors. New findings
in cancer research are presented each year at its annual conference.
Conference abstracts are posted on the ASCO web site.

Bonnie J. Addario Lung Cancer Foundation
www.thelungcancerfoundation.org
Phone 415-357-1278
c/o White Space, Inc.
601 4th Street, Suite 215, San Francisco, CA 94107
The Bonnie J. Addario Lung Cancer Foundation is focused on
research, early detection, education, prevention, and treatment.

CancerCare
Web site: *www.lungcancer.org*
Phone: 800-813-HOPE (4673)
A national nonprofit organization that provides free, professional support services to anyone affected by lung cancer. Services include counseling, education, financial assistance and practical help. Information is available in Spanish.

Joan's Legacy: Uniting Against Lung Cancer
Web site: *www.joanslegacy.org*
27 Union Square West, Suite 304, New York NY 10003
Phone: 212-627-5500
Joan's Legacy is a non-profit organization committed to fighting lung cancer by funding innovative research and increasing awareness, with a special focus on non-smoking related lung cancer.

Lung Cancer Alliance (LCA)
888 16th Street, NW, Suite 800, Washington, DC 20006
Phone: 800-298-2436
Web site: *www.lungcanceralliance.org*
LCA is the only national nonprofit organization dedicated solely to advocating for people living with lung cancer or at-risk for the disease. Programs include a toll-free hotline, phone buddy program, quarterly newsletter, and advocacy opportunities.

Lung Cancer Online Foundation (LCOF)
Post Office Box 762, East Setauket, NY 11733
Phone: 631-689-2754
Web site: *www.lungcanceronline.org*
LCOF is dedicated to improving the lives of people with lung cancer by providing information to patients and families via Lungcanceronline.org, a comprehensive, annotated directory to reliable lung cancer resources; and by directly funding lung cancer research.

LUNGevity Foundation
435 North LaSalle Street, Chicago, IL 60654
Phone: 312-464-0716
Web site: *www.lungevity.org*
LUNGevity is a nonprofit organization funding lung cancer research and providing support to the lung cancer community.

The Lung Cancer Caring Ambassadors Program
604 East 16th Street, Suite 201, Vancouver, WA 98663
Phone: 360-816-4186
Web site: *http://www.lungcancercap.org*
Through state-of-the-art information, awareness efforts, advocacy, and support, the Caring Ambassadors Lung Cancer Program (CAP Lung Cancer) is firmly committed to bettering the lives of people living with lung cancer and their loved ones.

National Cancer Institute (NCI)
NCI Public Inquiries Office, 6116 Executive Blvd., Rm. 3036A,
    Bethesda, MD 20892-8322
Phone: 800-4CANCER (NCI's Cancer Information Service)
Web site: *www.cancer.gov*
The NCI offers extensive up-to-date online and print information on lung cancer and its treatment, including clinical trials. Information is available in Spanish.

Cancer.Net
Web site: *www.cancer.net/portal/site/patient*
Oncologist-approved information for people with cancer, is maintained by the American Society for Clinical Oncology (ASCO).

National Lung Cancer Partnership
222 North Midvale Blvd., Suite 6, Madison, WI 53705
Web site: *www.NationalLungCancerPartnership.org*
Phone: 608-233-7905
The National Lung Cancer Partnership is the only national non-profit lung cancer organization founded by physicians and researchers, with

lung cancer survivors and advocates. Its mission is to decrease deaths due to lung cancer, and help patients live longer and better through research, awareness, and advocacy.

Print Publications

Henschke, C., et al. *Lung Cancer: Myths, Facts, Choices—and Hope*. New York: W. W. Norton, 2002.

Johnston, L. *Lung Cancer: Making Sense of Diagnosis, Treatment & Options*. Sebastopol, CA: O'Reilly & Associates, 2001.

CURE: Cancer Updates, Research & Education. Quarterly magazine that aims to explain scientific information to cancer patients. Print subscription is free to patients at *www.curetoday.com*.

Caregivers and Home Care

Family Caregiver Alliance
180 Montgomery Street, Suite 1100, San Francisco, CA 94104
Phone: 415-434-3388
Web site: *www.caregiver.org*
Caregiver resources include an online support group and an information clearinghouse. Information is available in Spanish.

National Family Caregivers Association
10400 Connecticut Avenue, Suite 500, Kensington, MD 20895-3944
Phone: 800-896-3650 | 301-942-6430
Web site: *www.nfcacares.org*
NFCA provides education, information, support, and advocacy services for family caregivers.

CAREGIVERS (Association of Cancer Online Resources)
Web site: *www.acor.org* (Click on "Mailing Lists" and then select "CAREGIVERS.")
Online discussion group for caregivers of cancer patients.

Guide for Cancer Supporters: Step-by-Step Ways to Help a Relative or Friend Fight Cancer (R.A. Bloch Cancer Foundation)
Web site: *www.blochcancer.org*

Print Publications

Houts, P. S. and Bucher, J. A., eds. *Caregiving: A Step-by-Step Resource for Caring for the Person with Cancer at Home.* Atlanta, GA: American Cancer Society, 2000.

Children

Kids Konnected
27071 Cabot Road, Suite 102, Laguna Hills, CA 92653
Phone: 800-899-2866 | 949-582-5443
Web site: *www.kidskonnected.org*
Provides extensive support resources and programs for children who have a parent with cancer.

Talking to Children—A Guide for a Parent with Cancer (CancerBACUP)
Web site: *www.cancerbacup.org.uk* (Enter "talking to children" in the search box.)

Print Publications

Harpham, W. S. *When a Parent Has Cancer: A Guide to Caring for Your Children.* Companion book: *Becky and the Worry Cup.* New York: Perennial Currents, 2004.

Clinical Trials Resources

There is no single resource for locating clinical trials for lung cancer. It makes sense to check repeatedly with all of the resources listed below because new trials are continually added. Clinical trials services are also emerging to help match patients to clinical trials. Some of these services can be useful for obtaining information and saving time, but it is important to read the company's privacy statement before using them and know whether the company is being paid for recruiting patients.

NCI Clinical Trials

Phone: 800-4CANCER

Web site: *www.cancer.gov/clinicaltrials/findtrials*

The National Cancer Institute (NCI) offers comprehensive information on understanding and finding clinical trials, including access to the NCI/PDQ Clinical Trials Database.

NIH/NLM Clinical Trials

Web site: *ClinicalTrials.gov*

Clinical trials database service developed by the National Institute of Health's National Library of Medicine.

Centerwatch Clinical Trials Listing Service

Web site: *www.centerwatch.com*

Listing of clinical trials, including trials sponsored by drug companies.

Clinical Trials Resources (Lungcanceronline.org)

Web site: *www.lungcanceronline.org/treatment–experimental/
    clinicaltrials/index.html*

In addition to linking to the major clinical trials resources listed above, Lungcanceronline.org provides links to NCI-designated cancer centers and hospitals with lung cancer programs that are likely to be conducting clinical trials in lung cancer. These sites can be contacted directly for information on available lung cancer trials. Links to some clinical trials services and directly to drug company trial information can also be found in Lungcanceronline.org's clinical trials section.

NCI Clinical Trials and Insurance Coverage

Web site: *www.cancer.gov/ClinicalTrials/insurance*

Excellent in-depth guide to clinical trials insurance issues.

Print Publications

Finn, R. *Cancer Clinical Trials: Experimental Treatments & How They Can Help You.* Sebastopol, CA: O'Reilly & Associates, 1999.

Mulay, M. *Making the Decision: A Cancer Patient's Guide to Clinical Trials.* Sudbury, MA: Jones and Bartlett Publishers, 2002.

Complementary and Alternative Medicine (CAM)

American Academy of Medical Acupuncture
4929 Wilshire Blvd., Suite 428, Los Angeles, CA 90010
Phone: 323-937-5514
Web site: *www.medicalacupuncture.org*
Professional site with articles on acupuncture, a list of frequently asked questions, and acupuncturist locator.

National Center for Complementary and Alternative Medicine (NCCAM)
Web site: *nccam.nih.gov*
Offers information on complementary and alternative medicine therapies, including NCI/PDQ expert-reviewed fact sheets on individual therapies and dietary supplements.

NCI Office of Cancer Complementary and Alternative Medicine (OCCAM)
Web site: *www.cancer.gov/cam/*
Information clearinghouse supporting the NCI's CAM activities.

Print Publications

American Cancer Society's Guide to Complementary and Alternative Cancer Methods. Atlanta, GA: American Cancer Society, 2000.

Kaptchuk, T. J. *The Web That Has No Weaver: Understanding Chinese Medicine.* McGraw-Hill, 2000.

Diet and Nutrition

American Institute for Cancer Research
1759 R Street, NW, Washington, DC 20009
Phone: 800-843-8114 | 202-328-7744 (in DC)
Web site: *www.aicr.org*
Supports research on diet and nutrition in the prevention and treatment of cancer. Provides information to cancer patients on nutrition and cancer, including a compilation of healthy recipes. Maintains a nutrition hotline for questions relating to nutrition and health.

Nutrition (American Cancer Society)
Web site: *www.cancer.org* (Enter "nutrition" in the search box.)
Nutrition resources include: ACS guidelines on nutrition, dietary supplement information, nutrition message boards, and tips on low-fat cooking and choosing healthy ingredients.

Drugs/Medications

MedlinePlus: Drug Information
Web site: *www.medlineplus.gov* (Click on the "drug information" button.)
Database with information on thousands of prescription and over-the-counter medications. Maintained by the National Library of Medicine.

Print Publications
Wilkes, G. *Consumer's Guide to Cancer Drugs*. Sudbury, MA: Jones and Bartlett Publishers, 2003.

Employment, Insurance, Financial, and Legal Resources

Americans with Disabilities Act (U.S. Department of Justice)
Web site: *www.usdoj.gov/crt/ada/adahom1.htm*
Provides information and technical assistance related to the ADA.

America's Health Insurance Plans (AHIP)

Web site: *www.hiaa.org/cons/cons.htm* (Click on "Consumer Information.")
Provides insurance guides for consumers. Topics include health insurance, managed care, disability income, and long-term care.

Cancer Legal Resource Center

Web site: *www.lls.edu/academics/candp/clrc.html*
919 S. Albany Street, Los Angeles, CA 90015
Phone: 866-THE-CLRC
A joint program of Loyola Law School and the Disability Rights Legal Center (formerly Western Law Center for Disability Rights). Provides information, educational outreach, and referrals to people with cancer who are facing legal problems related to their disease.

Centers for Medicare & Medicaid Services (CMS)
(Formerly the Health Care Financing Administration [HCFA])

Web site: *www.cms.hhs.gov*
The CMS is a Federal agency within the U.S. Department of Health and Human Services that oversees administration of:

- Medicare—federal health insurance program for people 65 years or older and some disabled people under 65 years.
  Phone: 800-MEDICARE
  Web site: *www.medicare.gov*
- Medicaid—federal and state health assistance program for certain low-income people.
  Web site: *www.cms.hhs.gov/medicaid/*
- Health Insurance Portability and Accountability Act (HIPAA)—insurance reform that may lower your chance of losing existing coverage, ease your ability to switch health plans and/or help you buy coverage on your own if you lose your employer's plan and have no other coverage available.
  Web site: *http://www.cms.hhs.gov/HIPAAGenInfo/*

Family and Medical Leave Act (FMLA)

Web site: *www.dol.gov/esa/whd/fmla/*

U.S. Department of Labor web page providing information about the Family and Medical Leave Act (FMLA).

Hill-Burton Program (Health Resources and Services Administration)

Phone: 800-638-0742 | 800-492-0359 in Maryland

Web site: *www.hrsa.gov/hillburton/*

Facilities that receive Hill-Burton funds from the government are required by law to provide free services to some people who cannot afford to pay. Information on Hill-Burton eligibility and facilities locations is available via phone or Internet.

Patient Advocate Foundation

700 Thimble Shoals Boulevard, Suite 200, Newport News, VA 23606

Phone: 800-532-5274

Web site: *www.patientadvocate.org*

Nonprofit organization helps patients to resolve insurance, debt, and job discrimination matters relative to their cancer diagnosis through case managers, doctors, and attorneys.

Social Security Administration (SSA)

Phone: 800-772-1213

Web site: *www.ssa.gov*

Oversees two programs that pay benefits to people with disabilities:

- Social Security Disability Insurance—pays benefits to you and certain members of your family if you have worked long enough and paid Social Security taxes.
- Supplemental Security Income—supplements Social Security payments based on need.

Veterans Health Administration

Phone: 877-222-8387 (Healthcare benefits) | 800-827-1000

Web site: *www.va.gov* (Click on "Healthcare" then "Health Benefits and Services.")

Eligible veterans and their dependents may receive cancer treatment and care at a Veterans Administration Medical Center.

Print publications

David S. Landry, *Be Prepared: The Complete Financial, Legal, and Practical Guide to Living with Cancer, HIV, and Other Life-Challenging Conditions*; New York, NY: St. Martin's Press, 1998.

Financial Assistance Programs

Air Care Alliance

Phone: 888-260-9707

Web site: *www.aircareall.org*

Network of organizations willing to provide public benefit flights for health care.

Finding Ways to Pay for Care
(National Coalition for Cancer Survivorship)

Web site: *www.canceradvocacy.org.* (Select "Find Resources" and then "Cancer Survival Toolbox.")

Partnership for Prescription Assistance

Web site: *www.pparx.org*

Coalition of drug companies and other groups to help qualifying patients get the medicines they need for free or very low cost through public and private programs.

Hospice and End-of-Life Issues

Growth House
Web site: *www.growthhouse.org*
Extensive annotated directory to hospice and end-of-life resources. Organized by topic.

Home Care Guide for Advanced Cancer (American College of Physicians)
Web site: *www.acponline.org/patients_families/end_of_life_issues/cancer/*
Guide for family and friends caring for advanced cancer patients who are living at home.

Hospice Net
Web site: *www.hospicenet.org*
Provides comprehensive information to patients and families facing life-threatening illness. Extensive resources addressing end-of-life issues from both patient and caregiver perspectives.

Patient Self-Advocacy Skills

Cancer Survival Toolbox (National Coalition for Cancer Survivorship)
Web site: *www.canceradvocacy.org* (Select "Find Resources" and then "Cancer Survival Toolbox.")
Topics include: communication skills, finding information, solving problems, making decisions, negotiating, and standing up for your rights. (Also available as audiotapes at 877-866-5748.)

Questions to Ask Your Doctor (Cancer.Net)
Web site: *http://www.cancer.net/portal/site/patient* (Enter "doctor questions" in the search box.)

Physician and Hospital Locators

Finding the Best Lung Cancer Care (*Lungcanceronline.org*)
Web site: *www.lungcanceronline.org/care/index.html*
Provides links to databases of lung cancer specialists (e.g., oncologists, thoracic surgeons) maintained by professional organizations and a listing of medical institutions that offer multidisciplinary lung cancer programs, including NCI-designated cancer centers.

Prevention and Risk Assessment

Cancer Research and Prevention Foundation
1600 Duke Street, Suite 500, Alexandria, VA 22314
Phone: 800-227-2732 | 703-836-4412
Web site: *www.preventcancer.org*
Offers information on prevention and early detection of cancer.

Your Cancer Risk (Harvard School of Public Health)
Web site: *www.diseaseriskindex.harvard.edu/update/* (Click on "cancer.")
Online assessment tool that estimates your lung cancer risk and provides tips for prevention.

Research Resources and Reference

Dictionary of Cancer Terms (National Cancer Institute)
Web site: *www.cancer.gov/dictionary/*

Medscape
Web site: *www.medscape.com*. (Enter "Lung Cancer" in the search box.)
Medscape is an excellent source for latest news in lung cancer research, including access to summaries of cancer conferences. Aimed at health care professionals. Registration required for free access to Medscape.

PubMed: MEDLINE (National Library of Medicine)
Web site: *www.pubmed.org*
Provides free online access to MEDLINE, a database of over 15 million citations to the medical literature.

Print Publications

Laughlin, E. H. *Coming to Terms with Cancer: A Glossary of Cancer-Related Terms*. Atlanta, GA: American Cancer Society, 2002.

Smoking Cessation

Quitnet

Web site: *www.quitnet.org*

Comprehensive web site for smoking cessation needs. Offers interactive personalized quitting tools, quitting guides, smoking cessation program locators, 24-hour online support/discussion, and links to smoking, tobacco, and cessation-related information and resources.

Smokefree.gov

Web site: *www.smokefree.gov*

Information and professional assistance for people seeking to quit smoking. Resources include cessation guides, telephone quitlines, instant messaging service, and print publications. Jointly sponsored by the National Cancer Institute, Centers for Disease Control, and American Cancer Society.

Support Services

Association of Cancer Online Resources (ACOR)

Web site: *www.acor.org* (Click on "Mailing Lists.")

ACOR offers online support groups for cancer patients. Lung cancer lists include: a general list (LUNG-ONC), and specific lists for small cell lung cancer (LUNG-SCLC), non-small cell lung cancer (LUNG-NSCLC) and bronchioloalveolar (LUNG-BAC). Also offers a wide variety of support groups for general and specific cancer- and treatment-related issues.

Cancer*Care*

275 Seventh Avenue, New York, NY 10001
Phone: 212-712-8080 | 800-813-4673
Web site: *www.cancercare.org*
Provides comprehensive support services and programs to people with cancer.

National Lung Cancer Partnership

222 North Midvale Blvd., Suite 6 Madison, WI 53705
Phone: 608-233-7905
Web site: *www.nationallungcancerpartnership.org*
Provides services under "Living with Lung Cancer", such as educational materials, inspirational stories and blogs, clinical trial information and an "ask the expert" section.

Phone Buddy Program (Lung Cancer Alliance)

Phone: 800-298-2436
Web site: *www.lungcanceralliance.org/facing/phone_buddy.html*
Offers peer-to-peer telephone support. Matches lung cancer survivors or their caregivers and family members with individuals who have faced, or are facing, similar circumstances.

R. A. Bloch National Cancer Foundation

4400 Main Street, Kansas City, MO 64111
Phone: 800-433-0464 | 816-932-8453
Web site: *www.blochcancer.org*
Provides Bloch-authored cancer books free of charge, a multidisciplinary referral service, and patient-to-patient phone support.

Vital Options International

15060 Ventura Boulevard, Suite 211, Sherman Oaks, CA 91403
Phone: 800-477-7666 | 818-788-5225
Web site: *www.vitaloptions.org*
Produces "The Group Room," a weekly, syndicated radio call-in show (with simultaneous webcast) covering important and timely topics in cancer. Previous shows are archived for access on the web site.

Wellness Community
919 18th Street, NW, Suite 54, Washington, DC 20006
Phone: 800-793-WELL | 202-659-9709
Web site: *www.thewellnesscommunity.org*
Provides educational programs and support groups for people with
cancer and their families.

Print Publications

Holland, J. C., and Lewis, S. *The Human Side of Cancer*. New York:
Perennial Currents, 2001.

Schimmel, S. R., and Fox, B. *Cancer Talk: Voices of Hope and Endur-
ance from "The Group Room," the World's Largest Cancer Support
Group*. New York: Broadway Books, 1999.

St. John, Tina M. *With Every Breath: A Lung Cancer Guidebook*,
2005. Presented by the Lung Cancer Caring Ambassador's
Program. Also available on-line at *www.lungcancerguidebook.org*.

Symptoms, Side Effects and Complications

Fatigue

CANCER-FATIGUE (Association of Cancer Online Resources)
Web site: *www.acor.org* (Click on "Mailing Lists" and then select
"CANCER-FATIGUE.")
Online discussion list covering cancer and treatment-related fatigue.

National Cancer Institute
Web site: *www.cancer.gov*
Phone: 800-4-CANCER

American Cancer Society
Web site: *www.cancer.org*
Phone: 800-ACS-2345

NCI/PDQ Fatigue

Web site: *cancer.gov* (Enter "fatigue" in the search box.)
Expert-reviewed information summary about cancer-related fatigue.

Print Publications
Harpham, W. S. Resolving the Frustration of Fatigue.
   CA: A Cancer Journal for Clinicians. 49 (1999): 178–189.
Outstanding article by a patient/physician discusses cancer-related
fatigue and how to deal with it.

Nausea and Vomiting

NCI/PDQ Nausea and Vomiting

Web site: *cancer.gov* (Enter "nausea" in the search box.)
Expert-reviewed information summary about nausea and vomiting
related to cancer and its treatments.

Nutritional Problems

NCI/PDQ Nutrition

Web site: *cancer.gov* (Enter "nutrition" in the search box.)
Expert-reviewed information summary about the causes and management of nutritional problems occurring in cancer patients.

Oral Complications

NCI/PDQ Oral Complications of Chemotherapy and Head/ Neck Radiation

Web site: *cancer.gov* (Enter "oral complications" in the search box.)

Pain

The National Pain Foundation (NPF)

3611 South Clarkson Street, Englewood, CO 80113
Web site: *www.painconnection.org*
NFP web site offers online education and support communities for
pain patients and their families, including cancer pain and palliative
care resources.

NCI/PDQ Pain

Web site: *cancer.gov* (Enter "pain" in the search box.)
Expert-reviewed information summary about cancer-related pain.
Includes discussion of approaches to the management and treatment
of cancer-associated pain.

Print Publications
Abrahm, J. L. *A Physician's Guide to Pain and Symptom Management
in Cancer Patients, 2nd ed.* Baltimore, MD: The Johns Hopkins
University Press, 2005.
Aimed at healthcare professionals, this practical and comprehensive
textbook is also an excellent resource for patients.

Peripheral Neuropathy

The Neuropathy Association
60 East 42nd Street, Suite 942, New York, NY 10165
Phone: 212-692-0662
Web site: *www.neuropathy.org*

CANCER-NEUROPATHY (Association of Cancer Online Resources)
Web site: *www.acor.org* (Click on "Mailing Lists" and then select
"CANCER-NEUROPATHY.")
Online discussion group for patients dealing with neuropathy induced
by cancer or its treatments.

Print Publications
Almadrones, L. A. and R. Arcot. "Patient Guide to Peripheral Neuropathy." *Oncology Nursing Forum* 26, no. 8 (1999):
1359–1362.

Pleural Effusion

Management of Pleural Effusion (CancerBACUP)
Web site: *www.cancerbacup.org.uk* (Enter "pleural effusion" in the
search box.)
Explains pleural effusion and its treatment.

Sexual Effects

CANCER-FERTILITY & CANCER-SEXUALITY
   (Association of Cancer Online Resources)
Web site: *www.acor.org* (Click on "Mailing Lists." and then
   select "CANCER-FERTILITY" and/or "CANCER-
   SEXUALITY.")
Online discussion lists about fertility and sexuality issues associated
with cancer.

NCI/PDQ Sexuality and Reproductive Issues
Web site: *cancer.gov* (Enter "sexuality" in the search box.)
Expert-reviewed information summary about factors that may affect
fertility and sexual functioning in people who have cancer.

Tests and Procedures

Cancer Imaging (National Cancer Institute)
Web site: *cancer.gov* (Enter "cancer imaging" in the search box.)

Laboratory Tests (MEDLINEplus)
Web site: *www.nlm.nih.gov/medlineplus/laboratorytests.html*

Print Publications

Margolis, Simeon, ed. *The Johns Hopkins Consumer Guide to Medical
   Tests: What You Can Expect, How You Should Prepare, What Your
   Results Mean.* Baltimore, MD: The Johns Hopkins University
   Press, 2001.

Treatment Information and Guidelines

NCI/PDQ Non-small Cell Lung Cancer Treatment & Small Cell Lung Cancer Treatment

Web site: *cancer.gov* (Enter "lung cancer" in the search box and then select "Lung Cancer Home Page.")

Expert-reviewed summaries about the treatment of NSCLC and SCLC.

Chemotherapy and You (NIH/NCI)

Web site: *cancer.gov* (Enter "Chemotherapy and You" in the search box.) Also available in print by calling 800-4CANCER.

Radiation Therapy and You (NIH/NCI)

Web site: *cancer.gov* (Enter "Radiation Therapy and You" in the search box.) Also available in print by calling 800-4CANCER.

Surgery for Lung Cancer (CancerHelp UK)

Web site: *www.cancerhelp.org.uk* (Enter "surgery for lung cancer" in the search box.)

Survivorship Issues

LT-SURVIVORS (Association of Cancer Online Resources)

Web site: *www.acor.org* (Click on "Mailing Lists" and then select "LT-SURVIVORS.")

Forum for discussion of issues of concern to long-term cancer survivors.

National Coalition for Cancer Survivorship (NCCS)

1010 Wayne Avenue, Suite 770, Silver Spring, MD 20910
Phone: 301-650-9127 or 888-650-9127
Web site: *www.canceradvocacy.org/*

Print Publications

Harpham, W. S. *After Cancer: A Guide to Your New Life*. New York: Perennial Currents, 1995.

Women and People of Color

National Women's Health Information Center
8270 Willow Oaks Corporate Drive, Fairfax, VA 22031
Phone: 800-994-9662
Web site: *www.4women.gov*

National Lung Cancer Partnership
222 North Midvale Blvd., Suite 6, Madison, WI 53705
Phone: 608-233-7905
Web site: *www.nationallungcancerpartnership.org*

Office of Minority Health
Post Office Box 37337, Washington, DC 20013–7337
Phone: 800-444-6472
Web site: *www.omhrc.gov*

Glossary

A

Adenocarcinoma: A type of non-small cell lung cancer; a malignant tumor that arises from glandular tissue.

Adjuvant therapy: Therapy given after initial treatment to increase its effectiveness; for example, adjuvant chemotherapy following surgery.

Advance directives: Legal documents that allow you to prepare for future medical possibilities and to assign someone to act on your behalf in the event you become unable to direct your own medical care.

Alopecia: Hair loss.

Alveoli: Tiny air sacs that compose the lungs.

Anemia: Low red blood cell count; may cause tiredness, weakness, and shortness of breath.

Angiogenesis: The formation of new blood vessels that allows tumors to grow.

Angiogenesis inhibitors: Drugs that prevent the formation of new blood vessels.

Antiemetics: Drugs that prevent nausea and vomiting.

Apoptosis: Process by which normal cells die when they are injured; often referred to as "programmed cell death."

Arms of a clinical study: Treatment group to which a patient is assigned in a RTC.

Asymptomatic: Without symptoms.

B

Benign: Not cancerous; not life-threatening.

Biopsy: Removal of tissue or fluid sample for microscopic examination.

Bone scan: An imaging test in which a radionuclear substance is injected into the veins and taken up by the bones in areas of potential metastatic disease.

Brachytherapy: Internal radiation therapy that involves placing "seeds" of radioactive material near or in the tumor.

Bronchioloalveolar carcinoma (BAC): A type of adenocarcinoma.

Bronchoscope: See **Bronchoscopy**.

Bronchoscopy: A procedure that involves inserting a flexible tube (**bronchoscope**) through the nose down into the lungs. Needles can be inserted through the bronchoscope to obtain biopsy samples.

C

Carcinogenesis: The development of cancer.

Carcinogens: Cancer-causing substances.

Cells: Microscopic units that make up the organs of the body.

Centigray: Unit of radiation; Same as a rad.

Central venous catheter (CVC): A thin tube that is surgically inserted to allow access to large veins.

Chemoprevention: The use of natural or synthetic substances to prevent cancer.

Chemopreventive agent: A natural or synthetic substance used to prevent cancer.

Chemotherapy: The use of medicine to treat cancer; a "whole-body" or systemic treatment.

Chromosomes: Strands of DNA and proteins in cell nucleus that carry units of heredity (genes).

Chronic obstructive pulmonary disease (COPD): Chronic bronchitis or emphysema.

Clinical trials: Research studies involving people.

Clubbing: A condition that causes the nails on the fingers to bulge out; clubbing occurs with many different types of lung problems.

Colony-stimulating factors: Substances that stimulate bone marrow to increase production of blood cells; also referred to as growth factors.

Complete blood count (CBC): A blood test that counts the number of white blood cells, red blood cells, and platelets.

Complete remission: The disappearance of all signs of cancer in response to treatment. This does not always mean the cancer has been cured. Also called **complete response**.

CT scan (computed tomography): Computerized series of x-rays that create a detailed cross-sectional image of the body.

Cranial irradiation: The exposure of the head to roentgen rays or other forms of radioactivity for therapeutic or preventive purposes.

Curative treatment: Treatment given with the intent to cure the patient of his or her cancer.

Cycle: The schedule of administration of chemotherapy which is repeated 4–6 times.

D

Deep vein thrombosis (DVT): A blood clot occurring in a deep-lying vein in the leg or pelvis.

Differentiation: A term used to describe the degree to which tumor tissue resembles normal tissue.

DNA (deoxyribonucleic acid): The "brain" of a cell; chromosomes are composed of DNA.

E

Electrolytes: Acids, bases, and salts essential for maintaining life; electrolyte abnormalities are imbalances of salts or chemicals in the blood.

Esophagus: The tube through which food travels from the mouth to the stomach.

External CVCs: IVs inserted in a large blood vessel. The other end is exposed through the skin and "capped off" so a patient does not have to carry an IV bag with them all the time.

F

Fibrosis: Scarring.

First-line therapy: Initial treatment.

Fraction: Single treatment of radiation. The total dose of radiation is usually given over multiple fractions.

G

Gene: Unit of heredity that regulates a particular function; located in a specific place on a chromosome.

Gene therapy: Treatment that replaces the abnormal gene in a cancer cell with a normal gene.

Grade: Term used to describe the degree to which tumor tissue resembles normal tissue.

Gray (Gy): Modern unit of radiation dosage. 100 rads is equal to one Gy.

Growth factors: Substances that stimulate cells to grow; drugs that help the bone marrow recover from the effects of chemotherapy (see also colony-stimulating factors).

Growth factor inhibitors: Substances that inhibit the growth factors that stimulate cells to grow.

H

Healthcare proxy: A person you have designated to make healthcare decisions for you in the event you become incapacitated.

Hematocrit: The proportion of the blood that consists of packed red blood cells.

Hemoglobin: The oxygen-carrying protein pigment in the blood, specifically in the red blood cells.

Hilar lymph nodes: Lymph nodes located in the region where the bronchus meets the lung.

Histology/histological: Tissue type; assessment of cellular features by microscopic evaluation.

Hospice: A philosophy of end-of-life care that focuses on palliative rather than curative care and provides a wide range of support to dying patients and their families.

I

Incidence: The number of new cases of a cancer (or any disease or event) in a defined population during a set period of time.

Informed consent: A process that provides potential participants in a clinical trial the information they need to make an informed decision about whether or not to participate.

Intensity Modulated Radiation Therapy (IMRT): A type of three-dimensional radiation therapy (3D-CRT) that uses radiation beams of varying strengths.

Interventional radiologist: A radiologist who uses x-rays and other imaging techniques to perform minimally invasive medical procedures.

Intravenous: In the vein.

L

Large cell carcinoma: A type of non-small cell lung cancer.

Ligand: An ion, a molecule, or a molecular group that binds to another chemical entity to form a larger complex.

Linac: A linear accelerator which produces high energy x-rays for radiation therapy.

Lobectomy: Surgical removal of a lobe of the lung.

Lobes: Clear anatomical divisions or extensions that can be determined without the use of a microscope (at the gross anatomy level). The right lung contains three lobes and the left contains two.

Lymph node: Small collections of white blood cells scattered throughout the body.

Lymph node dissection: Surgical removal of lymph nodes.

Lymphatic system: A vascular system that contains lymph nodes; cancer can spread through the lymphatic system.

M

Main stem bronchi: The two main breathing tubes (right main stem bronchus and left main stem bronchus) that branch off the trachea.

Main stem bronchus: One of the two main stem bronchi.

Malignant: Cancerous; cells that exhibit rapid, uncontrolled growth and can spread to other parts of the body.

Mediastinal lymph nodes: Lymph nodes located in the mediastinum, the area between the lungs.

Mediastinoscopy: A surgical procedure by which lymph nodes can be removed for microscopic examination.

Mediastinum: Area between the lungs.

Medical oncologist: A physician who performs comprehensive management of cancer patients throughout all phases of care; specializes in treating cancer with medicine.

Metastasis: The spread of cancer from the initial cancer site to other parts of the body.

Mini-thoracotomy: A type of minimally invasive chest surgery.

Mortality: The number of people who die of a disease.

Mutation: A damaged gene.

Myelosuppression: A decrease in the production of blood cells.

N

Nadir: Lowest measured value; period of low blood counts.

Negative margins: A phrase used when normal tissue is found at the edge of the biopsy sample.

Neoadjuvant therapy: Therapy given before the primary therapy; for example, neoadjuvant chemotherapy, which is sometimes given prior to surgery.

Neovascularization: Formation of new blood vessels that allows tumors to grow.

Neuropathy: See **peripheral neuropathy**.

Neutropenia: Low white blood cell count.

Neutrophil: A type of white blood cell that attacks bacteria.

Nicotine replacement therapy: Smoking cessation method that uses nicotine substitutes in various forms, including a patch, gum, inhaler, or nasal spray.

Non-small cell lung cancer (NSCLC): A type of lung cancer that includes adenocarcinoma, squamous cell carcinoma, and large cell carcinoma.

Nucleus: The center of the cell.

O

Oncogene: A gene that, when mutated, can allow a cell to grow uncontrollably.

Oncology nurse: A specialized nurse trained to provide care to cancer patients.

Oncology social worker: A social worker trained to provide counseling and practical assistance to cancer patients.

P

Palliation: Reducing symptoms.

Palliative care specialist: A physician trained in pain management.

Palliative treatment: Treatment given not with the intent to cure but with the intent to prolong survival and reduce symptoms from the tumor.

Pancoast tumor (superior sulcus tumor): A tumor occurring near the top of the lungs that may cause shoulder pain or weakness, or a group of symptoms including a droopy eyelid, dry eyes, and lack of sweating on the face.

Paraneoplastic symptoms: Symptoms that result from substances released by cancer cells and that occur at a site not directly involved with the tumor.

Parietal pleura: A membrane lining the chest wall.

Partial remission: A decrease in the size of a tumor, or in the extent of cancer in the body, in response to treatment. Also called **partial response**.

Passive smoking: Inhaling cigarette smoke of others.

Pathologist: A physician trained to examine and evaluate cells and tissue.

Patient-controlled analgesia (PCA): A method by which a patient can regulate the amount of pain medication he or she receives.

Performance status: The general condition of the patient.

Pericardial effusion: Accumulation of fluid inside the sac (pericardium) that surrounds the heart.

Pericardium: A double-layered serous membrane that surrounds the heart.

Peripheral neuropathy: Tingling, numbness, or burning sensation in hands, feet, or legs caused by damage to peripheral nerves by a tumor or by chemotherapy or radiation.

PET scan (positron emission tomography): A nuclear medicine imaging test that measures metabolism; can differentiate between healthy and abnormal tissue.

Phlebotomist: A technician trained to draw blood.

Photodynamic therapy (PDT): Treatment that uses laser light to kill cancer cells.

Placebo: An inactive substance (e.g., sugar pill). Placebos are rarely used in cancer trials.

Platelet: A type of blood cell responsible for clotting.

Pleura: A membrane surrounding the lung (visceral pleura) and lining the chest wall (parietal pleura).

Pleural effusion: Accumulation of fluid between the outside of the lung and the inside of the chest wall.

Pleural space: The area between the outside of the lung and the inside of the chest wall.

Pleurex catheter: Provides symptomatic relief of dyspnea related to recurrent pleural effusions.

Pleurodesis: A procedure to prevent recurrence of pleural effusion by draining the fluid and inserting medication into the pleural space.

Pneumonectomy: Surgical removal of the entire lung.

Pneumonia: An infection of the lung.

Pneumonitis: Irritation of the lungs.

Port: A type of central venous catheter that is surgically implanted under the skin.

Positive margins: A phrase used when cancer cells are found at the edge of the biopsy sample.

Prognosis: Predicted outcome; likelihood of survival.

Prophylactic cranial irradiation (PCI): Radiation to the brain with the intention of preventing the development of brain metastases.

Pulmonary embolism (PE): A blood clot that travels to the lungs causing full or partial blockage of one or both pulmonary arteries.

Pulmonary function tests (PFTs): A group of breathing tests used to determine lung health.

Pulmonologist: A physician who specializes in the diagnosis and treatment of lung diseases.

R

Rad: Unit of radiation.

Radiation fibrosis: Scarring of the lungs caused by radiation treatment.

Radiation oncologist: A physician who specializes in treating cancer with radiation.

Radiation therapy: Treatment that uses high-dose x-rays or other high energy rays to kill cancer cells.

Radiofrequency ablation (RFA): Treatment that uses high-frequency electric current to kill cancer cells.

Radioprotectant: A medication which reduces certain side effects of radiation.

Radiotherapy: The treatment of disease with ionizing radiation. Also called **radiation therapy.**

Randomized controlled trial (RCT): A research study in which the participants are assigned by chance (using a computer) to separate groups that compare different treatments; a method used to prevent bias in research.

Receptor: A protein molecule, embedded in either the plasma membrane or cytoplasm of a cell, to which a mobile signaling (or "signal") molecule may attach.

Red blood cell (RBC): The most common type of blood cell and the vertebrate body's principal means of delivering oxygen to the body tissues via the blood.

Regimen: Specific chemotherapy treatment plan involving the drugs, doses, and frequency of administration.

Rehabilitation specialist: A person trained to help patients recover from physical changes brought about by cancer or cancer treatment.

Remission: Shrinkage of tumor in response to treatment. May be either "complete" (total disappearance of tumor) or partial (the tumor has shrunk, but has not gone away entirely).

Resectable: Able to be surgically removed (resected).

Resection: Surgical removal.

Respiratory depression: Slowing of breathing.

Responding disease: Cancer which has shrunk in response to chemotherapy.

S

Schedule: How frequently chemotherapy is given.

Second-line treatment: Treatment method(s) used following an initial treatment that either does not stop cancer progression or stops it only temporarily.

Simulation: Planning the radiation fields with a CT scan.

Small cell carcinoma: A type of lung cancer that differs in appearance and behavior from non-small cell lung cancers (adenocarcinoma, squamous cell carcinoma, large cell carcinoma).

Small cell lung cancer (SCLC): Refers to small cell carcinoma, as opposed to non-small cell lung cancers (adenocarcinoma, squamous cell carcinoma, large cell carcinoma).

Sputum: Mucus and other secretions produced by the lungs.

Squamous cell carcinoma: A type of non-small cell lung cancer.

Stable disease: Cancer which has stopped growing following treatment.

Staging: Determining where the cancer is and how far cancer has spread.

Stent: A hollow tube that can be inserted via bronchoscopy into the airway to prevent it from being blocked or crushed by the tumor.

Stereotactic body radiotherapy: A highly precise radiation therapy technique; when used to treat brain metastases, it is called stereotactic radiosurgery.

Superior sulcus tumor: See **pancoast tumor**.

Superior vena cava syndrome (SVCS): A collection of symptoms that may include swelling in the neck, shoulders, and arms caused by a lung tumor pressing on the SVC, one of the large vessels leading into the heart.

Surgery: Removal of tissue by means of an operation (surgical procedure).

Systemic: Affecting the entire body.

T

Targeted therapy: Therapy directed at aspects of the cell that are specific for cancer.

Thoracentesis: A procedure that uses a needle to remove fluid from the space between the lung and the chest wall.

Thoracic surgeon: A surgeon who specializes in performing chest surgery.

Thoracotomy: A common type of lung surgery that requires a large incision to provide access to the lungs.

Three-dimensional conformal radiation therapy (3D-CRT): A type of radiation therapy that enables higher doses of radiation to be delivered more precisely than standard radiation therapy.

Thrombocytopenia: Low counts of platelets that may result in bruising and/or bleeding.

Trachea: Breathing tube (airway) leading from the larynx to the lungs.

Transthoracic (percutaneous) biopsy: A biopsy obtained by inserting a needle through the skin and chest wall into the tumor.

Treatment field: The area of the body which is radiated.

Tumor: A mass of tissue formed by a new growth of cells.

Tumor suppressor gene: A gene that can block cancer from developing.

V

VEGF (vascular endothelial growth factor): A sub-family of growth factors, more specifically of platelet-derived growth factor family of cystine-knot growth factors.

Video-assisted Thoracoscopic Surgery (VATS): A type of minimally invasive chest surgery.

Visceral pleura: A membrane surrounding the lung.

X

X-ray: High-energy radiation used to image the body.

W

Wedge resection: Surgical removal of the tumor and a small amount of lung tissue surrounding the tumor.

White blood cells: A type of blood cell which fights infection.

Index

Italicized page locators indicate a figure;
tables are noted with a *t*.

A

N

Nadir, 131
Nail care, 138
National Cancer Institute, 29, 98, 108, 163, 182, 192, 193, 197, 210
National Center for Complementary and Alternative Medicine, 114, 115, 201
National Coalition for Cancer Survivorship, 46, 205, 214
National Family Caregivers Association, 198
National Institute of Health, 114
National Institute of Health/National Library of Medicine Clinical Trials, 200
National Library of Medicine, 125
National Lung Cancer Partnership, 44, 48, 193, 197–198, 209, 215
National Pain Foundation, The, 211
National Women's Information Center, 215
Nausea, 79
    antiemetics and, 134
    chemotherapy and, 28, 73, 128
    information on, 211
    pain medications and, 151
    preventing, 75, 76, 80
Navelbine, 124, 132
NCCAM. *See* National Center for Complementary and Alternative Medicine
NCI. *See* National Cancer Institute
NCI Clinical Trials, 200
NCI Clinical Trials and Insurance Coverage, 200
NCI-designated cancer centers, 29
NCI Office of Cancer Complementary and Alternative Medicine, 201
NCI/PDQ Fatigue, 211
NCI/PDQ Nausea and Vomiting, 211
NCI/PDQ Non-small Cell Lung Cancer Treatment & Small Cell Lung Cancer Treatment, 214
NCI/PDQ Nutrition, 211
NCI/PDQ Oral Complications of Chemotherapy and Head/Neck Radiation, 211
NCI/PDQ Pain, 212
NCI/PDQ Sexuality and Reproductive Issues, 213
Needle sticks
    Emla and, 78
    IV, 75
Negative margins, 70
Neoadjuvant chemotherapy, 100
Neovascularization, 5

Neulasta, 131
Neupogen, 131
Neurontin, 139
Neuropathy, 14
Neuropathy Association, The, 212
Neutropenia, 129, 131
Neutrophils, 129
Nicotine addiction, 165
Nicotine replacement therapy, 164
N1, 21
Non-small cell lung cancer, 6
    chemotherapy recommendations and, 123
    curative treatment for, 63
    staging guidelines for, 21
    standard treatment options for, 98–105
        areas of research/clinical trials, 99–100, 103, 105
        Stage I & II, 98–99
        Stage III, 100–101
        Stage IIIA, 101
        Stage IIIB, 102–103
        Stage IV, 103–105
Non-small cell lung cancer-not otherwise specified, 7
Non-smokers, lung cancer diagnoses in, 49
Notebook or 3-ring binder, for medical information and paperwork, 39, 59
NSCLC. *See* Non-small cell lung cancer
NSCLC-NOS. *See* Non-small cell lung cancer-not otherwise specified
N2, 21
Nucleus, 3
Numbness, 139
Nurse practitioner, contact number for, 39
Nutrition, 46, 142, 170
    American Cancer Society's recommendations for, 162
    post-operative, 72
    resources on, 202, 211
Nutritionist, 28
N0, 21

O

Office of Cancer Complementary and Alternative Medicine (OCCAM), 114, 115
Office of Minority Health, 215
Oncogenes, 4
Oncologists, 29
Oncology nurses, 27, 39
Oncology social workers, 28
Opioids, 152, 153
Oral chemotherapies, 76
Oral complications, information on, 211

INDEX